World Religions for Healthcare Professionals

This third edition of a popular text introduces healthcare students and professionals to a wide range of health beliefs and practices in world religions. Chapters on various religions are written to offer an insider's view on the religion's historical development, key beliefs and practices, including ideas of health, sickness, death, and dying. The chapters include case studies and advice on what to do and what to avoid when caring for patients.

Introductory chapters invite the reader to consider the broad context of patient care in pluralistic society and explore one's personal orientation to others from different religions. How we care for patients from different backgrounds and cultures insists on professional boundaries that the reader may have not yet examined. A new chapter explores the relationship between religion and public health in light of the COVID-19 pandemic, asking the reader to consider what morally appropriate balance is required if and when personal faith conflict with public health needs.

Undoubtedly, the sensitivity with which clinicians communicate with patients and make decisions regarding appropriate medical intervention can be greatly increased by an understanding of religious and cultural diversity.

This is a core textbook for students studying healthcare, religion, and culture, and an invaluable reference for healthcare professionals.

Mark F. Carr, PhD, served as professor of ethics in the School of Religion at Loma Linda University and the theological co-director of the Center for Christian Bioethics at the same institution. He received his doctoral degree in religious ethics at the University of Virginia and wrote *Passionate Deliberation: Emotion, Temperance, and the Care Ethic in Clinical Moral Deliberation* (2001). After a brief time as chair of the Humanities and Social Sciences Department at Kettering College in Ohio, he now works in Anchorage, Alaska, where he serves as the senior director of ethics for Providence Health, Alaska.

Siroj Sorajjakool, PhD, received his degree from Claremont School of Theology in the field of personality and theology. For two decades he served as professor of religion, psychology, and counseling for the school of religion and, subsequently, professor in the department of counseling and family sciences for the school of behavioral health, Loma Linda University. He earned his second PhD in policy, management and educational leadership from Chulalongkorn University, Thailand. After returning to Thailand, he served as president for Asia-Pacific International University. He is currently professor of religion and theology at Asia-Pacific International University. His research interest focuses on exploring the issue of mental health within the Asian context and among ethnic minorities in Northern Thailand.

Ernest J. Bursey, PhD, is professor emeritus of religion in the department of Health and Biomedical Sciences at AdventHealth University in Orlando, Florida. He received his doctoral degree from Yale University in the field of New Testament studies with a dissertation, *Exorcism in the Gospel of Matthew* (1991). He has had a long career at Walla Walla University where he served as dean of the School of Theology, and more recently at AdventHealth University where he continues to teach undergraduate and graduate students in whole person care and world religions for healthcare professionals. He recently completed a commentary on the Book of Romans.

World Religions for Healthcare Professionals

Third Edition

Edited by Mark F. Carr, Siroj Sorajjakool and Ernest J. Bursey

Routledge
Taylor & Francis Group

LONDON AND NEW YORK

Designed cover image: © Getty Images

Third edition published 2024
by Routledge
4 Park Square, Milton Park, Abingdon, Oxon, OX14 4RN

and by Routledge
605 Third Avenue, New York, NY 10158

Routledge is an imprint of the Taylor & Francis Group, an informa business

© 2024 selection and editorial matter, Mark F. Carr, Siroj Sorajjakool, and Ernest J. Bursey; individual chapters, the contributors

The right of Mark F. Carr, Siroj Sorajjakool, and Ernest J. Bursey to be identified as the authors of the editorial material, and of the authors for their individual chapters, has been asserted in accordance with sections 77 and 78 of the Copyright, Designs and Patents Act 1988.

First edition published by Routledge 2009
Second edition published by Routledge 2017

British Library Cataloguing-in-Publication Data
A catalogue record for this book is available from the British Library

ISBN: 978-1-032-26564-3 (hbk)
ISBN: 978-1-032-26560-5 (pbk)
ISBN: 978-1-003-28886-2 (ebk)

DOI: 10.4324/9781003288862

Typeset in Sabon
by Newgen Publishing UK

Contents

Notes on contributors

Whitny Braun de Lobatón, PhD, is an assistant professor of ethics in the School of Religion at Loma Linda University as well as a clinical bioethicist and public health professional who specializes in the ethics of intercultural engagement in the healthcare setting. She is also a contributor to the *Huffington Post* and her work has been seen on the National Geographic Channel and heard on NPR. She was formerly the director of the Center for Jain Studies at Claremont School of Theology and has been active in the legal matter of the Jain death ritual of Sallekhanā before the Indian courts.

Ernest J. Bursey, PhD is Professor Emeritus of Religion in the department of Health and Biomedical Sciences at AdventHealth University in Orlando, Florida. He received his doctoral degree from Yale University in the field of New Testament studies with a dissertation, *Exorcism in the Gospel of Matthew* (1991). He has had a long career at Walla Walla University where he served as dean of the School of Theology, and more recently at AdventHealth University where he continues to teach undergraduate and graduate students in whole person care and world religions for healthcare professionals. He recently completed a commentary on the book of Romans.

Mark F. Carr, PhD, served as professor of ethics in the School of Religion at Loma Linda University and the theological co-director of the Center for Christian Bioethics at the same institution. He received his doctoral degree in religious ethics at the University of Virginia and wrote *Passionate Deliberation: Emotion, Temperance, and the Care Ethic in Clinical Moral Deliberation* (2001). After a brief time as chair of the Humanities and Social Sciences Department at Kettering College in Ohio, he now works in Anchorage, Alaska, where he serves as the senior director of ethics for Providence Health, Alaska.

Roy Kim, MD, is a staff physician at Riverside-San Bernardino County (California) Indian Health, Inc. He graduated from Loma Linda University School of Medicine and completed his family medicine residency at Florida Hospital in Orlando. He went on to a faculty development fellowship at Emory University's department of Family and Preventive Medicine, at which time he also received his Master of Public Health degree from Emory's Rollins School of Public Health. He has worked with the World Health Organization in Kosovo treating the Roma, Ashkali, and Egyptian Gypsy population. He has also tended to patients in Africa, Asia, Eastern Europe, and South America.

Douglas Kohn, Rabbi, MAHL, DD, is Senior Rabbi of Temple Beth Jacob in Newburgh, New York. He received his graduate and rabbinic training at Hebrew Union College-Jewish Institute of Religion, with rabbinic ordination in 1987, and Executive Leadership training at Northwestern University, Evanston, Illinois. Prior to his current position, he served as rabbi in Redlands, California, Hoffman Estates, Illinois, and assistant and associate rabbi in synagogues in Buffalo and Baltimore. He also served as an adjunct instructor for Hilbert College in Hamburg, New York. He is the editor of *Life, Faith, and Cancer: Jewish Journeys through Diagnosis, Treatment and Recovery* (2008), and *Broken Fragments: Jewish Experiences of Alzheimer's Disease* (2012).

Andy Lampkin, PhD, is professor of religion in the department of Health and Biomedical Sciences at AdventHealth University, in Orlando, Florida, where he teaches biomedical ethics at the undergraduate and graduate levels. He received his divinity degree and doctoral degree from Vanderbilt University, specializing in ethics and society, and the medical humanities. He has had a productive academic career teaching at Oakwood University and Loma Linda University. His current academic interests are on racial and ethnic health disparities, and the intersection of race, health care, and social justice. As an active scholar he has given numerous presentations, published several articles, and co-edited *African American Seventh-day Adventist Healers in a Multicultural Nation* (2021). As an engaged scholar he serves on Institutional Review Boards and Hospital Ethics Committees.

David R. Larson, DMin, PhD, is Emeritus Professor of Religion at Loma Linda university where he specialized for 46 years in theological and biomedical ethics while also teaching courses in philosophy, theology, world religions. Along with Jack W. Provonsha and James Walters, he was one of three Co-Founders of the university's influential Center for Christian Bioethics. He published many articles and several book chapters. He edited *Abortion: Christian Issues and Options* (1992), *Homosexuality: Some Seventh-day Adventist Perspectives* (2008) and *Making the Whole Person Whole: Papers and Presentations on Religion, Ethics and Medicine by Jack W. Provonsha* (2018). He received his DMin degree from Claremont School of Theology and PhD degree from Claremont Graduate University.

Arvind Mandair, PhD, is endowed professor of Sikh studies at the University of Michigan at Ann Arbor where he holds the SBSC chair in Sikh studies. He received his PhD in chemistry from Aston University in Birmingham, United Kingdom, and PhD in philosophy/Sikh studies from the University of Warwick, also in the UK. He is the author of *Religion and the Specter of the West: Sikhism, India, Postcoloniality and the Politics of Translation* (2009). He is the founding co-editor of the journal *Sikh Formations: Religion, Culture and Theory*, published by Routledge.

Hamid Mavani, PhD, is Associate Professor of Islamic Studies at Bayan Islamic Graduate School. His expertise in Islamic Studies stems from both academic training at Universities as well as specialized theological training at the traditional seminaries in the Muslim world. His primary fields of interest include Islamic legal theory and ethics, women and Shi'i law, Islam and secularity, intra-Muslim discourse, and environmental ethics. He is the author of a book published by Routledge in June 2013 titled, *Religious Authority and Political Thought in Twlever Shi'ism: From Ali to Post-Khomeini* and is co-author with Dr. Ahmad Kazemi-Moussavi of a work titled *Isamic Legal Methodology: A New Perspective* (2022). Dr. Mavani's scholarship also includes several academic articles and translations of Islamic texts from Arabic and Persian into English. In particular, the seminal work of the jurist, Dr. Mohsen Kadivar, titled *Blasphemy and Apostasy in Islam: Debates in Shi'a Jurisprudence*, trans. Hamid Mavani (2021).

Supaporn Naewbood, DrPH, is an assistant professor in nursing at Narasuan University, Pitsanulok, Thailand. She received her master's degree in health education from Chulalongkorn University, her second master's degree in community health nursing, and her DrPH from Mahidol University.

Julius J. Nam, PhD, JD, received his doctorate in religion from Andrews University where he wrote a dissertation on the relationship between Seventh-day Adventism and evangelical Protestantism in the United States. He has taught at Loma Linda University and Pacific Union College. He currently works for the US Department of Justice as an assistant United States attorney in Los Angeles, California.

Carla Gober Park, PhD, is vice president of wholeness & faith strategy at the corporate office of AdventHealth. Previously, she served as assistant vice president of spiritual life at Loma Linda University, director of the Center for Spiritual Life and Wholeness, and served on the teaching faculty of the School of Religion and the School of Medicine. She holds a bachelor's degree in religion and two master's degrees – one in public health education and the other in marriage and family counseling. As a registered nurse she served as a spiritual care nurse specialist and as a health educator. She received her doctoral degree in religious studies from Emory University where her focus was in the area of attachment, memory, and meaning.

Kwang-Hee Park, PhD, OMDLAC, received her doctoral degree in theology and personality from Claremont School of Theology and her doctorate in oriental medicine and acupuncture from South Baylo University in Orange County, California, where she worked as a researcher and patient counselor in the research department. She currently teaches both graduate courses in research, patient counseling, and psychology at South Baylo's department of Oriental medicine and herbology.

Manoj Shah, MD, is head of pediatrics gastroenterology division at Loma Linda University Medical Center and associate professor of pediatrics at Loma Linda University. He received his medical degree from Medical College, Baroda University in Gujarati, India and completed his residency at Cardinal Glennon Children's Hospital at St. Luke's Medical Center. He also served as vice president for the Federation of Gujarati Associations of North America, West Zone. He is the author of numerous peer-reviewed journal articles.

Siroj Sorajjakool, PhD, received his degree from Claremont School of Theology in the field of personality and theology. For two decades he served as professor of religion, psychology, and counseling for the school of religion and, subsequently, professor in the department of counseling and family sciences for the school of behavioral health, Loma Linda University. He earned his second PhD in policy, management and educational leadership from Chulalongkorn University, Thailand. After returning to Thailand, he served as president for Asia-Pacific International University. He is currently professor of religion and theology at Asia-Pacific International University. His research interest focuses on exploring the issue of mental health within the Asian context and among ethnic minorities in Northern Thailand.

Gerald R. Winslow, PhD, is the founding director of Loma Linda University's Institute for Health Policy and Leadership, and a professor of religion in the university's School of Religion. Previously, he served LLU as dean of the School of Religion, vice chancellor, and vice president for mission and culture. He received his undergraduate education at Walla Walla University and his master's degree at Andrews University. He earned his doctorate from Graduate Theological Union in Berkeley. He has also been a visiting scholar at Cambridge University, the University of Virginia, and the University of Tubingen. For over 40 years, he has specialized in teaching and writing about ethics, especially biomedical ethics. His current work focuses on the intersections of social and health policy. His books include *Triage and Justice* (1982) and *Facing Limits* (1992). His articles have appeared in academic journals such as *Western Journal of Medicine*, *Journal of Pediatrics*, *Hasting Center Report*, *Journal of Medicine and Philosophy*, and *General Dentistry*. He has presented seminars and lectures at universities and for professional groups throughout North America and in Australia, Europe, Russia, Africa, and Asia. He serves as the chairperson for Stakeholder Health's Advisory Council. He is also a member of the California Technology Assessment Forum, a public forum for the evaluation of new healthcare technologies. He has served as a consultant in biomedical ethics for major healthcare systems and for research conducted by pharmaceutical companies.

Preface and acknowledgments

This third edition of *World Religions for Healthcare Professionals* rolls off the press in 2023, in the wake of a pandemic. The provision of healthcare in America continues to undergo stresses and strains from virtually every direction imaginable, supply chain limitations, corporate financial struggles, caregiver burnout, staffing shortages, and unforeseen challenges that make for foundations that just keep moving beneath our feet. We, the editors and authors, hope that within this seeming chaos, the reader will remain focused on patients. Patients who are persons with stories and families and relationships that sustain and support them, often times embedded within their religious traditions.

Basic care offered to these patients, these persons, does not change all that much. Despite the swirl of current events, politics, and corporate shifting, the basic equation of caring for each other remains the core of healthcare and the core of this text. Among the elements of our present context, religion is also central. The pluralism that defines the United States becomes very real in the emergency rooms, hallways, surgical suites, and nursing units in the country's hospitals, clinics, and nursing homes. Young Jain physicians meet Evangelical Christian men and women in these encounters daily. Jewish patients cared for by Muslim nurses and physicians is common. Chinese Buddhist therapists help Roman Catholic mothers in home health services. Every imaginable combination of interaction and religion plays out in American healthcare every single day. It behooves us then to have some sense of who we are as caregivers and who our patients are. Religion and faith are indeed central to our work.

Despite the challenges of caring for each other, often as complete strangers, we commend to you the chapters within. For some of us, meeting people who may have very different life stories and religious traditions is difficult. When our broader culture seems to pour fire on our differences and conflicts, difficulties come right through to our conversations with patients and families. Others of us walk confidently into difficult conversations, regardless of the religious context. Patient–caregiver relationships can often be tense, sometimes escalating to verbal, even physical, violence. The understanding and appreciation caregivers can offer persons/patients may help deescalate tense situations in clinical care. This is especially so as it relates to our religions. Across the entire spectrum of the world's religions, treating others as you yourself would like to be treated (often referred to as the "golden rule") has existed for millennia. To be understood and to have one's religious beliefs known and respected is simply essential to how we care for each other.

We have carefully approached this project from a non-partisan perspective. In other words, we do not offer this book for North American Christians to learn more about non-Christians. Anyone who works in healthcare knows that as many, if not more, of the healthcare providers in North America are non-Christians. We do not need a book that looks out toward the Other from a Christian (or any privileged) perspective to see what they believe and who they are. The Hindu psychologist needs to know about Latter-day Saints as much as Catholic nurses need to know about Taoists. The Muslim surgeon needs to know about Jehovah's Witness beliefs as much as the Sikh pharmacist needs to know about her Jewish patient. The Shi'a public health official needs to know more about the Sunni family who lives just down the street.

We find these inter-religious conversations to be incredibly energizing and useful. Useful to a society that needs more recognition and appreciation of diversity. Useful to a community that purposefully seeks points of commonality while respecting points of difference.

Chapters 1 through 3 set the stage for entry into the specific chapters on the world's religions. After the initial three chapters, we have maintained a consistent chapter structure aimed at the reader's need for a useful reference to specific religions. After the *introduction* in each chapter, we thought it important to have some sense of the demographic footprint of the religion. Each author did their own research on demographics and naturally, since they did not all use the same sources, the reader may find some variation across the chapters. Our authors are experts in religion and healthcare, not demographics. Following the *demographics* section, a brief *history* of the religion fills out the preparation for a focused look at the *beliefs and practices* of the religion particularly as it relates to health and healthcare. These beliefs and practices are explored in three sub-headings: *general, health and disease, death and dying*. After the *conclusion* we include a short table of "*dos and don'ts*." The *case studies* included at the end of the chapter have proven to be a very engaging discussion opportunity for professors and students using this text. We include "*questions for reflection*" at the end of each case study. Finally, a glossary of key terms is available at the end of each chapter focused on a particular religion.

In addition to the individuality that each author brings to their chapter, this collection illustrates the fact that the study of religion may be an objective, scientific, and academic venture. And that it can be, simultaneously, highly personal. We consider this academic exploration both essential and enriching. But for those who may read this text from a lived experience of faith, taking an objective, scientific approach may be new and somewhat challenging. Ernest J. Bursey, in Chapter 1, walks the reader into the waters of such personal and professional space with the deftness that comes with decades of teaching experience.

In Chapter 2, Mark F. Carr and Gerald R. Winslow describe the interaction and methodological realities of ethics and religion/spirituality as patients (persons) are cared for. Hospital-based clinical ethics is intertwined with our sub-cultures and religions. And in the hospital context ethics have a direct bearing on how religion/spirituality is lived out. Carr and Winslow focus on the ethics of caregiver–patient interaction with specific regard to religion and spirituality.

Chapter 3 is new to this third edition and was inspired by the experience of the COVID-19 pandemic. The chapter, *Religion and public health*, seeks to shine a light on the interface of Religion, Health, and the Public's Health. Andy Lampkin and Mark F. Carr have long engaged students on this interface of public health and religion. The pandemic revealed the intricacies of our interwoven sub-communities in pluralistic societies. Our faith and religion compel innumerable influences in our daily lives, both privately and publicly. Our life in society compels innumerable adjustments and compromises for the good of the whole. The local, state, and federal regulations and laws aimed at enhancing the public's health sometimes conflict with our religious convictions. These conflicts need to be carefully navigated and we are all part of that equation. How can public health officials engage and interact with our religious communities in positive ways to protect and enhance our health and the common good?

Chapters 4 through 13 focus attention on specific world religions particularly relevant to the context of healthcare. Two things are impossible in our effort here, namely, representing all of the world's religions as well as capturing the full range of lived realities within each of the religions presented in this volume. There is a wide range of beliefs and practices under the umbrella of each religion. We cannot possibly capture the full range of expression for each. These two impossibilities have not kept us from moving forward into the learning conversation.

We wish to acknowledge the special support and help we have received from those in classrooms who are using this text. Of note are the case studies found in this edition. The first edition did not include case studies. The second edition included case studies and now this third edition contains even more. We are of the opinion that case studies are powerful methods in the learning venture. Short of living through the event, when truly embraced as a thought experiment with robust discussion, it forces our imagination beyond typical patterns. Those of us who have used this textbook in academic coursework find high pedagogical value in using the case studies to talk through some of the biases we all bring to the topic.

At the end of each case, we noted our colleagues who submitted the case studies for our use and we offer acknowledgment and appreciation for their help; the text is better because of them. Regarding our case studies work, special appreciation is due to Dr. Garret Potts of the Department of Religious Studies at the University of South Florida whose help teaching, editing, and focusing these cases has been invaluable. He and Dr. Ernest J. Bursey both work with a special interfaith group who also find discussions of cases to be meaningful to our pursuit of the common good and the public's health. Interfaith America www.interfaithamerica.org/, formerly known as Interfaith Youth Core, has been a helpful resource for us as these cases were developed.

Mark F. Carr, Anchorage, Alaska

1   Introduction

Ernest J. Bursey

Welcome to world religions from a healthcare perspective. The study of world religions offers you an added resource in meeting the needs of your patient and clients because you will possess a more accurate knowledge of their religious beliefs and practices.

Extensive research supports the claim that patients who actively participate in a religion enjoy a longer life span and shorter stays in hospital than do their counterparts. The *Handbook of Religion and Health*, 2nd ed. estimates that over 2100 qualitative studies have been published, most indicating a positive correlation between religion and health (Koenig et al. 2012). A particularly important finding for our purposes is that the health benefits from religious affiliation are not restricted to one specific religion.

Since 1965 the number of patients with religious affiliations other than Christianity has significantly increased because the general population of the United States has become more religiously diverse. That year President Lyndon Johnson signed the Immigration and Nationality Act that ended the national quota system that had discriminated against persons from Asia and the Middle East. As a result of this legislative change, immigrant believers of the typically Asian religions increased in the US. According to the 2018 General Social Survey, 6.2% of Americans identify with a religion other than Christianity (Burge 2021: 27).

One positive benefit from the study of world religions is a better understanding of the growing number of immigrant healthcare professionals who actively embrace a faith tradition other than Christianity. In the years since 1965, preferential access in immigration to the United States has been given to applicants with scientific and medical expertise needed in the United States. As a result, physicians affiliated with a religion other than Christianity are disproportionately represented compared to the percentages in the general population. Results from a 2005 national survey of physicians showed that collectively, Jewish, Muslim, Hindu, and Buddhist physicians amounted to 23% of the responses (Curlin et al. 2005). Nearly all of my graduate nursing students report working alongside nurses or physicians who openly hold to a faith other than their own and who believe their faith makes them better healthcare professionals.

Hopefully as a result of reading this volume you will become more aware of the religious minorities in your own community and perhaps more sensitive to the challenge they face in maintaining their religious practices and culture. The majority of legal immigrants continues to be Christian since the largest percentage of immigrants to the United States are from Central and South America. But significant numbers of Hindus and Muslims, particularly from South Asia, have immigrated and become naturalized citizens. Mosques and temples sprout up in suburban American neighborhoods to meet the religious needs of this growing population. Funding for these projects is underwritten in part by affluent

DOI: 10.4324/9781003288862-1

immigrant professionals including those in healthcare and engineering. At the dedication of a new temple in Florida on June 15–19, 2005, a souvenir booklet itemized the names of donors; out of a total of 77 named devotees contributing $10,000 or more each, 42 were listed as "Dr.," with ten couples listed as double "Drs." (Hindu Society of Central Florida 2005).

On a wider front, your knowledge about the religions of the world here in the United States will give you one more window into understanding current events. Thirty to forty years ago, futurists predicted that organized religions would wither away under the advance of secularism. They were wrong. People today are still likely to identify with ancient religious traditions.

Personal benefits and challenges

We are more than healthcare professionals. We are, first, human beings who share with all human beings, including our patients, the mysteries of existence, the common experience of suffering, and the certainty of death. As creatures with a bent to find meaning in our lives we seek to cope with events that seem to defy and rationalize explanation. The medical explanation of an immediate cause for the death of a child falls short of explaining why we are living in a universe where this can happen. Religious people, like all people, seek to find a conceptual framework that accounts for and even counters the apparent randomness of events. Religions attempt to answer the fundamental questions of why we have been born, the purpose of our existence, and what, if anything, lies beyond this life. It is true that when we study another religion we are confronted with strange terms and even stranger practices that may give us the feeling that we are studying the beliefs of aliens quite different from ourselves. But at a deeper level, studying the religious beliefs of faiths other than our own may give us a sense of the deep bond we share with all other persons. Any medical care that fails to give homage to this common humanity dishonors the dignity of those it seeks to serve.

If you consider yourself an adherent of a particular religion you may sense the inherent challenges, and even risks, in studying other religions. Students often discover they were misinformed about what a particular religion teaches, as a result of taking a course on world religions. Occasionally an introductory course in world religions leads to further study into a new religion and even the change of religious affiliation. A former student described being required as a child to attend her parents' church where she never felt at home with the ritual and preaching. She confessed to me, "I often wanted to run out screaming." When she was an adult student in a world religions course she chose to visit a Buddhist retreat center where she felt embraced within the serene setting and calmed by the instruction in meditation that reduced her inner stress. She called me from 2500 miles away to announce that she had found her true spiritual home. Her case is an exception. Much more often students challenged in a course in world religions decide to look more closely at their own religious tradition and acquire a more accurate knowledge of its basic beliefs. As any teacher of world religions can attest, most Americans, regardless of the religious tradition to which they belong, have a limited understanding of the resources of their own religion. It has often been observed that by learning a second language a person develops a more acute understanding of one's native language. Likewise, a course in world religions often serves as a catalyst for a more mature grasp of a childhood faith.

While most healthcare professionals welcome the opportunity to better understand the religious perspectives of their clients and colleagues, not all are persuaded of the need to spend time, effort, and expense to study the various world religions. First, some are deeply convinced that their own faith is the only true one and that other religions teach dangerous ideas that can lead to the embrace of error, perhaps with eternal consequences. Often persons holding this position also see it as their duty to share their beliefs with others, out of both a sense of responsibility and a concern for the welfare of others. Upon reflection, it becomes clear that any realistic attempt at sharing one's faith requires a sound knowledge of the beliefs and practices of the other. All persuasion begins on common ground. Given that the social decorum of healthcare professionals demands appropriate restrictions upon sharing one's faith, healthcare professionals living with a mandate to share their faith may live with an inner tension between the demands of their faith and their profession. Nonetheless, devout caregivers who await opportunities to speak of their faith are more likely to find receptive hearers if they are knowledgeable about the others' beliefs.

A second group that may be resistant to investing in the study of world religions are those who describe themselves as non-religious. They are occasionally very aware of the harmful effects of dogmatism and superstition. Yet concern for their patients' well-being may lead them to learn enough to avoid the pitfalls that would offend a devout patient. A study of the world views and distinctive practices outside of the narrow healthcare arena may seem irrelevant to the curriculum of a healthcare professional. It must be admitted that the non-religious or secular population is typically under-represented in courses on world religions. Perhaps you are part of that group. This marginalization masks the evidence that the secular or non-religious segment of American society, while still small, is growing in numbers and voice. Openly acknowledging the presence and the viewpoints of non-religious students is a vital step toward greater dialogue and engagement over the influences of religion.

What is a world religion?

Ask ten people on the street for a definition of religion and you may get ten different answers, some focusing on the beliefs, some on practices or rituals. Even when scholars define religion the results can be quite diverse, depending in part on whether a scholar is a sociologist or a psychologist, an anthropologist, or a theologian. If the sociologist stresses the communal nature of religious practice and the social construction of religious beliefs, the psychologist may address religion within the individual's search for autonomy and personhood. The anthropologist stands outside the circle of religious belief in describing myth and ritual within a specific cultural context, while the theologian presumes the possibility of communication with a supernatural reality. For the purposes of this book, rather than hammering out a definition of religion, we focused on identifying and comparing the features that are common to different religions and how they interface with healthcare in the United States.

Where do I come from? Why am I here? Why am I ill, in pain, and suffering? What happens after death? Religion can be understood as a response to these questions of human origin, purpose, and well-being, especially in the light of the certainty of death and the uncertainties of life. The mystery of our own existence and the realization that we are transient creatures attracts many to religions that claim access to the unseen beyond the senses. Each day we are immersed in a stream of events that arrive without warning. Religions typically offer the believer some sort of coherent framework of meaning to interpret these apparently random events. Religions also issue guidance on how we may order our daily lives through the observance of times of worship, prayer, reading of sacred texts, and meditation.

The focus of this volume is the so-called "world religions," although Native American religions and new religious movements are included. Humans are universally religious. Yet not every religion can be called a world religion. When academics refer to world religions the list typically includes Hinduism, Buddhism, Islam, Judaism, Taoism, Confucianism, and Christianity. Other religions occasionally included are Yuruba, Sikhism, Jainism, Zoroastrianism, and the Baha'i. Shinto, the national religion of Japan, and nature religions such as Wicca may be included as well. In addition to being widespread, the so-called "world religions" typically possess scriptures or religious texts that serve to anchor religious beliefs and written collections of authoritative teachings that can be transmitted from one generation to the next. Jews revere the Tanakh and study the rulings of rabbis found in the Mishnah and Talmud. Muslims consider the Qur'an to contain the very words of Allah and draw on the preserved rulings of legal scholars familiar with the collections of sayings about and by Muhammad. But humans have been religious long before they learned to transmit knowledge through the medium of writing. Throughout the world and on every inhabited continent indigenous peoples have feared unseen spiritual forces and sought to control them or seek their favor, often by elaborate ritual and the observance of taboos.

Religion and culture

This textbook focuses on the beliefs and practices that are characteristic of religions, not on culture and cultural practices. But religion is a part of culture. Culture includes the totality of the customs and practices of a distinct group of people. So, separating what is religious from what is cultural is not an easy matter. It might seem that the beliefs and rituals of a world religion like Buddhism or Islam or Christianity ought to be the same anywhere in the world. Yet the way a religion is practiced varies considerably from culture to culture, and age to age. Labels like "fundamentalist," "conservative," "progressive," and "liberal" are used to describe the variations within a religion. These variations may not be isolated but part of a larger reality of how religion manifests itself all across the world.

Deciding what belongs under the umbrella of religion can be complicated and confusing. Persons living in one country may include rituals or customs as part of their religious obligation that persons of the same religion in a different country consider optional or even refuse to practice. For instance, the practice of female genital mutilation or female circumcision is widely practiced in Egypt. The Egyptian Demographic and Health Survey reported that 86% of Egyptian women have undergone some form of female circumcision (United Nations Population Fund 2022). The Egyptian government made the procedure illegal in 2008, with severe penalties for doctors performing the procedure. Yet the practice persists. A frequently cited reason is the belief that good Muslim women undergo the operation. In contrast to the societal encouragement in Egypt, the conservative Muslim society of nearby Saudi Arabia looks down upon the practice as against the principles of Islam. Saudi Arabia has legally forbidden the procedure as well. Another misperception is that the practice is limited to Islamic religion/cultures, which is untrue. Christians living in the same cultures engage in similar practices (United Nations Population Fund 2022).

Who then decides whether a belief or practice is to be truly considered a religious obligation or simply a traditional cultural practice? In some religions, a recognized religious authority may make the decision about what is core and non-negotiable. Roman Catholics generally consider the decisions of the Magisterium (the teaching office of the Church headed by the Pope) to define what they are to believe and practice. In some religions, there may be no comparable universal recognized figure or authoritative group.

The impact of American culture on transplanted faith traditions is often profound. Immigrants who come to the United States from a country where their religion was sponsored by the government discover on arriving that if they want to retain their religious faith, they must take more personal initiative than they had taken in their country of origin. The openness and even secularization of American culture can have a double edge effect on religious minorities, on the one hand leading to a deepening personal understanding of one's faith, but on the other hand raising legitimate concerns about the religious commitments of the second and third generation. I recall a Muslim businesswoman from Tanzania telling the students in my classroom that she knew more about her faith and why she was a Muslim than her relatives in Tanzania where their religion was taken for granted and supported by loudspeakers announcing the times of prayer.

Scholars of religions in America note that transported religions, including even the major world religions, tend to morph into more distinctly American forms. The openness of American culture makes isolation difficult. A continual infusion of new immigrants ensures the retention of traditional practices and views. But over time, something uniquely American or Westernized begins to emerge. Factors that drive this on-going process include the expectation of American women to fully participate and even lead out in religious functions, the constitutional freedom to openly discuss and debate religious matters, the recognized absolute right of personal choice in matters of faith, and the acceptance of inter-faith marriages. Debates over the physical presence of women in public worship continue to percolate in traditional Muslim and Orthodox Jewish communities.

The desire of immigrants to lessen prejudice by blending into the cultural landscape and to demonstrate loyalty to an adopted country leads to changes in the practice of their religion. RH Seager sees the emergence of an indigenous American Buddhism, though the process is far from completed (Seager 2002: 118).

More than a hundred years ago Japanese farmers immigrated to America, bringing their Shin Buddhism with them. Over time temples were built that outwardly imitated the appearance of Protestant churches unlike the traditional architecture of Shin Buddhist temples in Japan. Pews replaced mats. Western musical instruments, hymns, and even choirs were incorporated into the religious services. After the Japanese attack on Pearl Harbor in 1941 and President Roosevelt's executive order to round up citizens of Japanese descent, the name, Buddhist Mission of North America, was changed to Buddhist Churches of America (www.buddhistchurchesofamerica.org/about-bca).

The process of religious accommodation remains complicated. Many American converts to Buddhism pursue personal goals through solitary meditation practices. On the other hand, incoming immigrants from several Buddhist majority countries strive to maintain communal expressions of Buddhism while making concessions to American culture in part to retain the next generation. (*Pluralism Project* n.d.)

Not to be overlooked is the growing influence of beliefs and practices from immigrant religions particularly relevant in healthcare. Payment for Chinese acupuncture is widely, if not universally, accepted by health insurance plans. Mindfulness, part of the Eightfold Path of Buddhism, is securely embedded in hospitals and university research centers as a therapy for stress and stress related illness. The impetus to introduce Buddhist mindfulness practice into secular American healthcare using non-religious vocabulary is credited to Jon Kabat-Zinn, former Professor of Medicine at the University of Massachusetts. Faith-based hospitals in the Christian tradition have occasionally resisted what has been described as "stealth Buddhism" (Brown 2014). Yoga to improve one's health is now as American as apple pie, notwithstanding protests from Hindu purists and some fearful Abrahamic traditions.

Religion, ethics, and transformation

While religions have traditionally focused on how we ought to relate to the divine, all the major religions of the world also promote moral codes of conduct about how we relate to each other. Whether you look in the Jewish Tanakh, the Christian New Testament, the Buddhist Dhammapada, the Hindu Bhagavad Gita, or the Muslim Qur'an, these codes of conduct are quite similar in forbidding murder, adultery, stealing, lying, disrespect of parents and elders, etc. The Golden Rule attributed to Jesus in the New Testament, "Do to others what you would want them to do to you," can be paralleled by the words of Muhammad, Buddha, and other religious teachers. Some Americans fear that basic moral standards will be undermined by the growing number of the population that embrace non-Christian religions. Such fears are groundless. Religions of the world place high value on honesty, unselfishness, marital faithfulness, and the responsibility to preserve human life. Religious persons of every stripe tend to oppose abortion or the practice of active euthanasia at higher rates than more secular persons.

All the major religions of the world also address the contradictions of human behavior in our routine failure to uphold our own moral codes, frequently falling far short of basic human decency. These lapses require both an explanation and an antidote. The religions of the world tend to diverge from one another in their diagnosis of the cause for that gap between acceptable standards and actual moral conduct. It is not surprising that differing etiologies to account for moral failure leads to divergent prescriptions or strategies for closing the moral gap. Hindus and Buddhists expect reincarnation or rebirth to deal with negative karma accumulated from wrongdoing in previous lives. Muslims practice the regiment of submissive prayer five times daily as an aid to keeping their mind on the straight path of righteousness. Christians hold to the benefits from a crucified Savior to counter the consequences of a fatally flawed human nature.

The rise of the "nones"

The percentage of Americans claiming no religious affiliation rose dramatically from 16% in 2008 (when the first edition of this textbook appeared) to 29% in 2021 (Smith 2021). A closer look reveals important differences among these "nones." Most retain a belief in a God of some sort. But every category shows a trend away from organized religion (Lipka 2016). This trend appears to follow the pattern of European secularization. Some find no interest or value in the discussion or practice of religion. In 2014 one in ten

Americans simply had no interest in religion. Age comparisons are even more alarming to those who see religious belief as a bulwark of human moral behavior. While two-thirds of those born before 1946 claim religion to be important in their lives, the numbers for those born between 1981 and 1996 drops to only four out of ten (Gjelten 2015). Efforts to understand and counter these trends are evident in every faith tradition.

Factors affecting the drop in religious affiliation include a sense that science conveys truth while religion peddles tradition, disbelief in the relevance of religious organizations, publicized moral corruption of religious leaders, and, in the case of Christianity and Islam, rejection of an angry or vengeful God. The plurality of religions can create a disbelief that any of them can claim to provide the exclusive avenue to the Divine.

Recent surveys suggest that as many as one in four Americans now self-identify as "spiritual but not religious" (SBNR). Often, they "have rejected a God stereotyped as a judgment overseer and instead have substituted the idea of a sacred force which is impersonal and benevolent" (Mercadante 2014: 230). A self-declared former SBNR, Mercadante predicts that many will in time move from the category of "none" to affiliate with a religion. The search for a coherent meaning to human existence, for rituals that counteract a self-centered spiritual experience, and for the strength that comes from belonging may lead them to a religious community. Ideally, that community will portray a loving God and offer a counter view to the values of a market-driven culture.

Surveys as recent as 2019 suggest that 4% of Americans considered themselves atheists, more than double the percentage in 2007; while self-identified agnostics also almost doubled at 5% in 2014. Two out of three atheists are males with a median age of 34 compared with a median age of 46 for the general public. Deep suspicion of atheists shows up with 51% of Americans in 2014 viewing atheism as a personal deterrent when voting for the President in 2014, down from 63% in 2007. Recently the strident calls of prominent atheists like Richard Dawkins and Christopher Hitchens to eliminate religious belief and abolish religious privileges have found a widespread audience. But other atheists recognize the social value of religion and seek to establish corresponding non-theistic or humanist communities that can work with religious organizations in bettering human life (Krattenmaker 2016).

Finally, a secondary parallel trend deserves mention, the shift among professed Christians from denominational affiliation to the more generic designation of "non-denominational Christian," which more accurately represents a shift to evangelical Protestantism.

Religion and healthcare

One of the distinctive features of this textbook on world religions is the focus on healthcare. Historically, virtually all religions have been concerned with illness and the maintenance of health. Some offer explanations for the presence of sickness and death. Some paradigms for treating illness are theoretically tied to specific religions. Ayurveda, a form of medical care widely practiced in India and to some extent in North America as an alternative to Western medicine, is closely associated with Hinduism. Traditional Chinese medicine, including acupuncture and moxibustion, has theoretical roots in Taoist thought. On the other hand, the missionary religions of Buddhism, Christianity, and Islam have not been so closely tied to precise medical paradigms, but their followers have accommodated to a variety of medical practices.

For thousands of years religion has been involved in bringing physical and mental healing. Illness has been widely considered as caused by negative or even hostile spiritual forces that need to be appeased or even banished in order to restore health. Jesus, the founder of Christianity, healed the sick, often by means of exorcism, alongside his preaching. His enemies attributed his particular effectiveness as an exorcist to an alleged alliance with Satan. A key factor in the spread of Christianity was the perceived effectiveness of Christian missionaries in banishing evil spirits in the name of Jesus. Yet today physicians in the west who call themselves Christians typically do not include demonic possession as a diagnosis. The hospitals in AdventHealth, a faith-based Christian healthcare system with the motto, "Extending the healing ministry of Christ," do not have departments of exorcism but follow the protocols of Western biomedical healthcare. Yet many devout believers continue to put their confidence in prayers and rituals to address what they consider to be the spiritual causes of their illness. Whether or not you hold such views, you will need to become aware of the differing understandings of illness to assist your patients more skillfully in their recovery.

The rapid growth of medical knowledge has raised profound challenges to the ethical norms of all the world religions. Religious leaders have struggled to keep up in providing the faithful with guidance regarding life-creating, life-extending, and life-denying technologies that were previously unimaginable but now are readily available. Rather than automatically embracing the latest medical technological advance, religious leaders show hesitancy, even skepticism. Shall sperm donors be denounced as adulterers? Does *in vitro* fertilization blur the distinction between the Creator and the human creature? Is the circulation of blood through external cleansing equipment during surgery a violation of the Bible's prohibition against ingesting blood?

If God is the source of human life, under what circumstances then, if any, may a pregnancy be terminated? Muslim and Catholic theologians differ on when an embryo receives a soul or is deemed a person. Consequently, regarding female use of contraception, they issue different rulings about drugs or procedures that may impede the development of a conceptus. When is the removal of artificial life support justified? Religions typically place a high value on human life and stand almost united against active euthanasia and physician assisted suicide. Yet limits to the utilization of life-extending technology must be drawn somewhere. In most religions the authority of a religious leader will be recognized by only a portion of the faithful and so conflicting views may be offered as options. The Orthodox Jewish believe that the soul of a person gradually withdraws from and remains with the body after brain function stops; this may infuse tension between medical personnel and the dying person's family. These conflicts make graphic headlines in newspapers eager to boost reader interest: "Catholic godson of woman on life support fights to get proxy back" (Saul 2014), "Hasidic boy in legal fight over life support buried" (Furse 2008). Chayim Aruchim (n.d.), a program of the ultra-conservative Agudath Israel of America, appeals to Jews to seek the guidance of a rabbi trained in Jewish law or halakha when navigating end of life issues. For a comprehensive guide to the range of Orthodox halakha reasoning see Shabtai (2012). Less conservative Jews in the Reformed and Conservative branches of Judaism are more likely to end life support when no brain activity can be detected, and the beating heart is dependent on a mechanical ventilator.

The importance of preserving the body intact for a future resurrection of the deceased has often stood in the way of Muslims, Jews, and Catholics families granting permission for medical autopsy for potentially valuable medical knowledge. Autopsy itself has seemed to some to be like the desecrating of the fallen warrior on the field of battle, forbidden by the sacred text of the Qur'an. Yet when organ transplantation offered the gift of life to persons dying from organ failure, theologians and religious leaders reconsidered long held positions and took up the questions of when organs could be harvested, who should receive them, etc. When the faithful accept the gift of an organ for the sake of preserving their own lives, fairness calls for reciprocity by allowing them to offer that gift to another person.

A recommendation to enhance your learning

This text was carefully prepared by knowledgeable experts to offer you a reliable overview of several recognized world religions. Yet I recommend that you supplement a careful reading of this text with face-to-face conversations with persons from other religious traditions who are active in the practice of their own religion. No other experience better awakens your awareness of what you will read in the pages ahead.

Reading a chapter in this book about a religion other than your own will serve to introduce you to that tradition. It would require years of careful study and experience for a Christian, for instance, to know the vast range of views and practices that are held among Hindus. Should you interview a person from another religious tradition you may discover that this person holds views about their religion that differ somewhat from what you read in the chapter. On the other hand, if you read the chapter carefully before the interview, you may learn something about their religion that they themselves did not know. Most important, you will learn from them how someone else actually practices the religion they love. That is a treasure worth seeking.

Conclusion

As you study each of the religions, picture in your mind four concentric circles. In the outer and largest circle you will find the basic information about a world religion. Then picture inside that larger circle a smaller circle to represent how that religion is practiced here in the United States. The inevitable impact of American culture produces accommodations and innovations in each religion. Conversely, a diversity of religions enriches American culture. In this textbook you will find some attention to this circle of cultural immersion. Likely you will find further evidence of accommodation if you take up the suggestion of interviewing a person from another religious tradition.

Now envision a still smaller circle to represent American healthcare. Here the religious beliefs and practices of patients and healthcare practitioners interact with one another. When faced with health issues, patients from every religion draw strength from it. A significant part of every chapter will be spent considering that inner circle of the intersection of healthcare and religion. Finally, you can imagine an even smaller circle to represent your own thoughts, ideas, and perhaps convictions about religion.

Studying and working in the field of healthcare prompts one to see that we are living in a time of change. Buddhist, Christian, Hindu, and Muslim healthcare professionals are caring for patients of all faiths and denominations in American hospitals and clinics. The tides of change continue to flow. Will we learn how to work together with our cultural and religious differences? Will we be able to hold on to our old exclusionary ideas of "us" and "them?" Or will we make larger inclusive circles of commitment and care that respect and even value this religious diversity? Your study of world religions from a healthcare perspective will give you the confidence you need to join the larger circle.

Case study #1: finding common ground

A 15-year-old boy accompanied by his mother presented to the Emergency Room with shortness of breath and chest pain. The medical team suspected, based on preliminary tests, that the young man had suffered a descending aortic aneurysm. He was transferred to the pediatric cardiovascular intensive care unit.

A nurse concerned for the well-being of the boy's mother asked if there was any one she could call on her behalf to support her. She politely declined and said, "I have no one." Overwhelmed with sympathy, the nurse asked if she might call a hospital chaplain to be with her. The mom reluctantly acquiesced.

The chaplain introduced herself and asked more about the boy lying in his bed. The mother, visibly uncomfortable, said, "I do not believe in God, I am an atheist, so I am not sure what you can do for me." The chaplain stayed silent for a minute and then responded, "I am respectful of your beliefs, I am here because if I were in your situation, I would want someone with me."

Questions for reflections

1. What did the nurse have in mind when she called the chaplain to provide support? What assumptions are likely present behind the mother's statement, "I am not sure what you can do for me"?
2. Why might the mother acquiesce, albeit reluctantly, to the offer of a chaplain's visit? What could the chaplain provide for an atheist mother other than overt religious words and services? What might be involved in "someone to be with me"?
3. What are the common human needs, fears, and hopes that atheists share with other human beings who believe in God and some form of afterlife?

Submitted by Jocelyn Shaw

Case study #2: finding common ground

Annie was a 51-year-old Buddhist female hospitalized after a flare up of her multiple sclerosis. Her lungs were failing. Ginny, her mother, was daily at her daughter's bed-side. A nurse recognized an underlying tension between mother and daughter, so she asked for a chaplain with a knowledge of Buddhism to visit. It became evident that Ginny, a devout Christian, was concerned about Annie's salvation. Annie felt that her mother did not accept her conversion to Buddhism and resisted her mother's efforts to pray together.

The chaplain briefly retold the story of the Buddha, beginning with his teaching of *The Four Noble Truths*. Then they talked about how Buddha was willing to sacrifice his life as he tried to find a way out of suffering (*dukkha*) for humanity. Turning to Ginny, the chaplain noted that five centuries later, another teacher, Jesus, offered himself as the way out of suffering for humanity. Then the chaplain asked if they could meditate together and then express their gratitude to each other for the gift of compassion that moves the world toward goodness. With tears, mother and daughter expressed their gratitude.

Later, the chaplain returned with a book written jointly by two world renowned religious leaders, one Buddhist and the other Christian. The three read a few pages together before the chaplain had to visit elsewhere. Ginny continued reading aloud to her daughter. Annie died on the following day.

Questions for reflection

1. Evaluate the chaplain's efforts to help Ginny and Annie bridge their differences without directly addressing the mother's concern for her daughter's salvation. What was most helpful in removing the barriers between Annie and her mother?
2. The chaplain sought to provide spiritual care for both the mother and her daughter in part by presenting some similarities between Buddha and Jesus, particularly as they sought to address human suffering. What do you think of this approach?
3. Would you characterize the chaplain's approach as pluralist, inclusivist, or exclusivist? How would you characterize your own view?

*Submitted by Oleg Kostyuk

Bibliography

Brown, CG. (2014) "Mindfulness: Stealth Buddhism for Mainstreaming Meditation?" *The Huffington Post*. December 2, 2014, updated February 1, 2015. www.huffingtonpost.com/candy-gunther-brown-phd/mindfulness-stealth-buddh_b_6243036.html

Burge, RP. (2021) *The Nones: Where They Came, Who They Are, and Where Are They Going*. Minneapolis, MN: Fortress Press.

Chayim Aruchim (n.d.) *Center for Culturally Sensitive End-of-Life Advocacy and Counseling*. https://chayimaruchim.com/

Curlin, FA., Lantos, JD., Roach, CJ., Sellergren, SA., and Chin, MH. (2005) "Religious Characteristics of U.S. Physicians: A National Survey," *Journal of General Internal Medicine*, 20(7): 629–634.

Egypt Demographic and Health Survey (2014) *Cairo, Egypt and Rockville*. Maryland, USA: Ministry of Health and Population and ICF International. http://dhsprogram.com/pubs/pdf/FR302/FR302.pdf

Furse, JH. (2008) "Hasidic Boy in Legal Fight Over Life Support Buried," *New York Daily News*, November 17, 2008. www.nydailynews.com/new-york/brooklyn/hasidic-boy-legal-fight-life-support-buried-article-1.339093

Gjelten, T. (2015) "Poll Finds Americans, Especially Millennials, Moving Away from Religion," *The Two Way: Breaking News from NPR*, November 3, 2015. www.npr.org/sections/thetwo-way/2015/11/03/454063182/poll-finds-americans-especially-millennials-moving-away-from-religion

Hindu Society of Central Florida (2005) *Maha Kumbabhishekam and Prathistapana Celebrations, June 15–19, 2005, Souvenir and Directory*. Casselberry, FL: Hindu Society of Central Florida. www.orlandohindutemple.org/

Koenig HG., King DE., and Carson VB. (2012) *Handbook of Religion and Health*, 2nd ed. New York, NY: Oxford University Press.

Krattenmaker, T. (2016) "The 'Nones' Are Becoming Somethings," *Reflections Yale Divinity School*, Spring, 2016: 44–45. https://reflections.yale.edu/article/all-together-now-pluralism-and-faith/nones-are-becoming-somethings

Lipka, M. (2016) "Ten Facts About Atheists," *Pew Research Center*, June 1, 2016. www.pewresearch.org/fact-tank/2016/06/01/10-facts-about-atheists/

Mercadante, LA. (2014) *Belief Without Borders: Inside the Minds of the Spiritual but not Religious*. New York, NY: Oxford University Press.

Pluralism Project (n.d.). "One Buddhism? Or Multiple Buddhisms?" Harvard University https://pluralism.org/buddhism

Saul, J. (2014) "Catholic Godson of Woman on Life Support Fights to Get Proxy Back," *New York Post*, March 20, 2014. http://nypost.com/2014/03/20/catholic-godson-of-woman-on-life-support-fights-to-get-proxy-back/

Seager, RH. (2002) "American Buddhism in the Making," in Prebish, CS. and Baumann, M. (eds.) *Westward Dharma: Buddhism beyond Asia* (pp. 106–119). Berkeley: University of California Press.

Shabtai, D. (2012) *Defining the Moment: Understanding Brain Death in Halakah*. New York, NY: Shoresh Press.

Smith, G. (2021) "About Three-in-Ten U.S. Adults Are Now Religiously Unaffiliated." *Pew Research Center*. www.pewresearch.org/religion/2021/12/14/about-three-in-ten-u-s-adults-are-now-religiously-unaffiliated/

Stedman, C. (2013) *How an Atheist Found Common Ground with the Religious*. Boston, MA: Beacon Press.

United Nations Children's Fund (2014) "Female Genital Mutilation/Cutting: What might the future hold?" *UNICEF*, New York https://data.unicef.org/resources/female-genital-mutilation-cutting-might-future-hold/

United Nations Population Fund (2022) "Female Genital Mutilation." https://egypt.unfpa.org/en/node/22544

2 From conceptual to concrete

Mark F. Carr and Gerald R. Winslow

Some people are more inclined to broad, theoretical views of life while others are more concerned with the practical matters and particular details of everyday life (Jonsen 1991: 14–16). Both patterns of thought are essential in religion and healthcare. The methods of decision making and patient care detailed in this chapter take this into account. Nationally and internationally, these two modes of thought are associated with two methods of clinical ethics decision making in healthcare. Principles-based reasoning, or what has come to be called principlism, as well as case-based reasoning, or casuistry, are both highly influential in the field of ethics and morality in healthcare decision making.

Principles-based patient care

There are four "pivotal moral principles" that are widely accepted as essential to establish an "analytical framework of general norms" in morally appropriate patient care. *Respect for autonomy, beneficence, nonmaleficence*, and *justice* have emerged from centuries of religious, social, and cultural attention to ethics. The institutions of our civilization have been significantly shaped by shared conceptions and applications of these four principles. Though there is debate about exactly how many principles suffice to capture the essence of this common morality, with some arguing for as many as seven, the most influential advocates of principlism assert that these four are sufficient (Beauchamp and Childress 2019: 13–25).

Before proceeding to a discussion of how the principles may be applied in the clinical setting, it will be helpful to provide a brief definition for each of the four:

- *Respect for autonomy*: respecting the choices of the patient. In recent decades, especially starting in the 1970s with the promulgation of the "Patients' Bill of Rights," much greater emphasis was placed on the ethical importance of honoring the patient's expressed values and decisions.
- *Beneficence*: ensuring the patient receives significant benefit from healthcare interventions. Patients generally trust their professional caregivers to give priority to the good of the patient over other potentially competing concerns. Seeking the patient's good is what the healthcare professions, in their codes of ethics, all profess.
- *Nonmaleficence*: guarding against harming the patient. One of the most time-honored commitments of healthcare professionals is captured in an oft-repeated Latin expression – *primum non nocere* – which means "first of all, do not harm."

DOI: 10.4324/9781003288862-2

- *Justice*: treating patients equitably, without unfair discrimination. The essence of this principle is a commitment to human equality with differences in treatment based on morally relevant considerations.

According to the most prevalent view of principlism, the four principles are not hierarchical; they are not to be considered in rank order since one is no more or less important than the others. Rather, they move in and out of relevance in any given case as details of the case are discovered and capture our attention. Based upon the case details, typically one of the principles will have greater practical significance than the others. The careful work of figuring out which of the principles should take priority in any particular case is the responsibility of caregivers and the people for whom they are caring. Let us illustrate:

A two-car accident involving a 24-year-old male alone in his vehicle and a family of five in a minivan brings out the paramedics. Upon arrival at the scene the family is found to have only minor injuries, but the young man has passed out from shock primarily due to a compound fracture of his left femur. He has lost a lot of blood. Paramedics do their best to revive him, and upon further assessment they believe that he probably also sustained a number of internal injuries. They rush him to the emergency room (ER) while trying to contact his family.

As principles-based reasoning goes, thus far in the case the paramedics have correctly responded under the principle of beneficence; they clearly are doing good for the patient, trying to keep him alive. Doing good for persons in distress is an immediate, intuitive, and also learned response for both lay and professional people in our society. In the ER, these beneficent responses are well established. Thus, it would seem rather odd, given this brief case description, for anyone in the emergency setting to appeal to other principles, such as justice. Nor is anyone likely to wonder if we are actually harming this young man (nonmaleficence). Since he is unconscious, it would also be nonsensical to ask him for his informed consent under the principle of respect for autonomy.

Imagine, however, that the details of the case shift rather quickly. Within the next couple of hours, the man's wife and extended family arrive at the ER with his advance healthcare directive in hand. The directive clearly indicates that he does not want any blood products in the event of a serious accident or critical illness. This is because he is a Jehovah's Witness and he holds religious convictions that forbid the use of blood products for medical care.

Within the next hour of treatment in the ER, the young man's condition continues to decline. While the fracture and associated bleeding are managed, the internal bleeding continues. His wife and family refuse to give consent for surgery, again citing the use of blood products. After considerable argument between the ER physicians and the family (the patient was still unconscious), the physicians and hospital administrators decide to seek a court order to allow them to take the young man to surgery and use the full measure of blood products and methods at their disposal. Thus, the hospital risk management team takes a request to the judge on call in the hope of getting an injunction that will allow them to use blood products. The judge rules in favor of the patient's family, thus effectively giving priority to respect for the patient's autonomy as expressed through his advance directive.

Principles-based reasoning is again at work here. One of the important reasons for an advance healthcare directive is to respect the personal choices of patients. Of course, these personal choices are often deeply influenced by a person's religion and spirituality. Thus, respect for autonomy comes to the fore as an important principle to consider in this specific case at this specific time. In light of the patient's religious desire to avoid the use of blood, the principle of beneficence is now in conflict with the principle of respect for autonomy. Additionally, if the ER team was simply to override the family's desire to follow his advance directive, one could argue that they would actually be harming the patient, thereby breaking the principle of nonmaleficence (avoiding harm) in the process.

While the family members are clear that they do not want their loved one to die, they do not want to override his clearly expressed religious convictions. And with frustrated reluctance, the ER team accepts the judge's decision to honor the young man's advance directive. There will be no surgery without the family's consent, and the ER must not use any blood products in caring for the young man. Despite their best efforts, the young man dies within the hour following the judge's decision.

The process of specifying, weighing, and balancing the four principles is a crucial skill in the principles-based method of caring for patients (Beauchamp and Childress 2019: 17–24). Critical thinking skills and self-reflective practices are essential tools for any clinician seeking to care appropriately for patients. It is part of clinicians' professional responsibility to evaluate the relevance of each of the principles and determine which of them will take priority over the others at any given point in the case. For nearly four decades, through eight editions of *Principles of Biomedical Ethics*, the four principles remain widely influential.

Closely associated with principlism is another prominent method of attending to religion and morality, referred to as "casuistry" or the "four-box" method. For ease of memory, we refer to it as "case-based" as it is compared and contrasted to the principles-based approach.

Case-based patient care

In their book, *Clinical Ethics*, proponents of the case-based approach, Albert Jonsen, Mark Siegler, and William Winslade, offered their model in deliberate contrast to the principles-based approach (Jonsen et al. 2021). The subtitle of their widely used book, "A Practical Approach to Ethical Decision Making in Clinical Medicine," already tells the reader much about the intention of their case-based mode of reasoning. The goal is to help healthcare professionals in the clinical setting come to ethically appropriate decisions in a way that attends to the most salient details in the most efficient way. To accomplish this, the authors describe four crucial factors of a case: (1) the medical conditions, (2) the patient's preferences, (3) the patient's quality of life, and (4) contextual features such as family dynamics, legal constraints, religious community, and financial resources that may influence decisions about care for the patient. The authors depict these four considerations in a four-quadrant table, with medical conditions and a patient's preferences in the upper two quadrants, and quality of life and contextual features in the lower two quadrants. Early on, the authors expressed the belief that most cases could be resolved almost entirely within the medical conditions quadrant, followed by sequential progression through the other three quadrants, as described earlier. Eventually, however, the proponents modulated this sequential, four-box approach in the direction of giving more holistic attention to the entirety of the quadrants. At the back of their book, they have even provided a removable card-stock page in order to facilitate having the four quadrants, with their accompanying questions, readily available to caregivers.

Given the pragmatic and often fast-paced context of inpatient care, the case-based approach gained popularity with physicians and other healthcare professionals when treating complex cases, including those in which the patient's religion represents a significant consideration. For busy clinicians, the focus on coming efficiently to decisions about individual cases has obvious appeal. The hefty, in-depth volume of the *Principles of Biomedical Ethics* makes it the more likely preference of professors and philosophers of medical humanities and ethics. While both publications express respect for religious convictions and diversity, neither of them gives extensive attention to religion and spirituality. Beauchamp and Childress (2019) argue that religion and spirituality are so pervasive throughout the entirety of our common morality that treating them as standalone topics might be misleading. Jonsen, Siegler, and Winslade, on the other hand, simply embed religion in their fourth box, "Contextual Features," with the following question: "Are there religious factors that might influence clinical decisions?" (Jonsen et al. 2021).

When resolving difficult clinical cases, including those with significant religious factors, healthcare professionals will be well-served by either method described. It is worth noting that the proponents of both the principles-based and the case-based approaches have incorporated some of the more persuasive elements of the others' arguments. This signals the value of employing a combination of methods in what some refer to as "reflective equilibrium" (Rawls 1971: 20). This expression, coined by philosopher John Rawls, points out the reality that our reasoned judgments, guided by established principles, are routinely adjusted by the specific details of any given case (Beauchamp and Childress 2019: 439–444). In similar fashion, our understanding of principles matures over time as we gain experience in their application to specific cases. In essence, this argument says that justification for a normative position taken in response to a religious or ethical quandary is found in the reasoning of both principles-based and case-based methods. The two are better understood as complementary rather than as competitors. If we were to study the patterns of case-based ethical decision making over time, it would likely reveal underlying principles like those asserted by Beauchamp and Childress. Identifying the principles and making them explicit facilitates the likelihood of shared understanding by those engaged in the decisions. Clear enunciation of the principles also enhances the orientation of new members of the caregiving team regarding the basis for ethical decisions.

There are three additional approaches to clinical ethics that need careful consideration if we are to create a comprehensive and ethically effective response to religious and spiritual concerns in the clinical setting. We address these under the rubrics of *narrative ethics*, *virtue ethics*, and *care ethics*. The additional insights and practical guidance from these approaches have considerable value in the clinical care of patients.

Narrative ethics

Have you ever asked someone a clear and pointed question only to have her or him respond by telling a story? A former student referred to being angry at her father when she was young because every time she asked him a hard question, he would sit back and tell her a story. She never really understood, until she heard the description of narrative faith and ethics. This approach features the central importance of stories – stories that form the essence of our religion, ethics, and spirituality. These are not limited to an individual's own personal stories, but they may also be the stories of one's family, community, church, school, state, nation, and so forth. Human beings are so deeply embedded in such stories that it would be impossible to resolve religious and moral dilemmas in ways that do not attend to the stories that shape the involved person's understanding of the context.

People hear, interpret, and repeat meaningful stories every day. Among the most powerful of these are the religious stories that thoroughly shape the lives of billions of people. Without the story of Siddhartha, what would Buddhism be? Without Muhammad, how would we understand the story of Islam? Christianity without Jesus is unthinkable. And lest anyone think this approach works only for religion, we might ask what of the United States of America, without George Washington? Or the Republic of South Africa without Nelson Mandela? Stories are powerful in shaping individual conscience and also influencing the social consciousness of entire societies.

Hilde Lindemann Nelson identifies at least five things we do with stories that may profoundly affect how we live our lives: (1) *reading* stories, (2) *telling* stories, (3) *comparing* stories, (4) *analyzing* stories, and (5) *invoking* stories. All five of these, according to the author, are part of the process of making sense of life (Nelson 1997: x–xii). In the realm of health and illness, it is often the case that the power of religious and spiritual stories is dramatically enhanced. It is hard to overstate the thoroughgoing nature of this approach to life and religion. One scholar who has focused on narratives in medical contexts, Kathryn Montgomery Hunter, insists that "narrative is the primary way of organizing and communicating" what it means to be human in our world. At the "heart of human knowing" lies an "interpretive process integral to shaping and understanding" our lives through story (Hunter 2004). Indeed, from this perspective, religion is unintelligible without thoroughgoing engagement in telling stories.

Young people may often be bored or annoyed with having to sit through the stories their parents or grandparents tell, some of which may be told over and over again. Yet, as those same young people themselves grow older, they often find themselves remembering and perhaps even recounting the same stories. Whether or not it is realized, the subconscious effects of stories shape the way we live and function in the world.

Often the intention of telling religious stories is to lead the hearers (or readers) to accept practical lessons. "Now boys and girls, the moral of the story is . . ." is the oft-used transition away from the details of the story itself to the lessons that children are supposed to learn from the story. Narrative religionists are prone to point out that the stories, in and of themselves, are strong enough to convey the lessons. There is no need to moralize at the end of the story. A crucial task for responsible humans, who share a concern for enhancing the spiritual and religious lives of their community, is simply to tell the stories well (Hauerwas and Jones 1989: 158–190).

In clinical care, much may be learned about patients by listening attentively to their stories. In particular, when patients near the end of their lives, families often need to retell the stories that have been important to them through the years. As much as possible, caregivers may help provide time for this process. Additionally, those caring for dying patients and their family members can use stories to foster understanding about what is happening in the dying process.

Attending to patients' life stories is an essential part of respecting them as persons. This means giving careful attention to a patient's self-understanding and goals of self-governance, which is essential in order to respect their *autonomy*. Listening to family stories about their religion and the proper practice of it near the end of life brings ongoing meaning in family life.

The focus on narrative highlights the personal roles of the participants in the story. The actors in the story portray characters of a certain sort. Almost any story has "good guys" and "bad guys" – persons with virtues and persons with vices. This realization leads us to turn to "virtue" or "character-based" approaches to religion and ethics.

Virtue ethics

The way of virtue is usually intimately connected to religion and spirituality, though it is true that one need not be either to be virtuous. Religion and spiritual practices have shaped or misshaped human character traits more effectively throughout history than most other human institutions. One of the ways virtues are fostered is through the practice of upholding exemplars to emulate. Within the world's prominent religious traditions there are typically appeals to moral and religious exemplars. Indeed, it would be impossible to imagine Christianity without Jesus, Islam without Muhammad, or Buddhism without Siddhartha. Those of us charged with imbuing the religious values and convictions of a faith tradition use reinforcing techniques to encourage our children to behave as our religious heroes have in the past. And again, this sort of reinforcement method is not limited to religion. Some of us are old enough to remember the *Nike* brand shoe commercials featuring the great basketball player Michael Jordan, that said simply, "I want to be like Mike" (Sommers and Sommers 2004: 209–276).

This character-based approach has bearing on both sides of any clinical scenario in which religion is an important factor. The patient and the patient's family and friends do well when they practice the virtues of courage, insight, openness, and vulnerability. Similarly, there are key virtues that caregivers practice so as to provide the best possible healthcare to patients and their families. According to physician-philosopher Edmond Pellegrino, fortitude, compassion, integrity, practical reason, and self-effacement, among others, are essential to remain true to the history of both healthcare and religion (Pellegrino and Thomasma 1993). To single out one virtue prevalent in religious communities that is essential to caregiving in our view, we will highlight altruistic compassion.

Virtues are not easily developed or perfected. Some believe that our personal character traits are primarily genetic rather than habits to be learned, practiced, or perfected. Character traits like open-mindedness or stubbornness seem to be things we come by naturally, whereas virtues like compassion and courage are qualities we may learn and practice over time (Borba 2002). Indeed, at the outset of learning a virtue like courage, we may have to fake it (Herdt 2008: 23–32). In a stressful situation, we may be frightened, but external observers might not be able to see that about us. Internal motivation and disposition are essential to the authentic exercise of the virtues. An external observer cannot tell when they see me engage in an apparently compassionate act whether or not I am actually compassionate. Indeed, given the complexity of human motivations, I may not be entirely certain about myself. A duty-based perspective on the life of faith stresses that one engages in an act that God or the gods have demanded. When I compassionately help an old person across the street, you may see me as a virtuous person, but I may simply be doing my duty according to my interpretation of what God requires. This is not the way of virtue. The way of virtue calls for personal authenticity and consistent, practiced intention to care for others out of the compassion in one's heart and soul. Habituating such character is the way of virtue, and often religion is part and parcel of any such habituation.

There are many influences of personal development for those seeking religious and character growth in the way of virtue. Genetic heritage may certainly make a difference. So also, one's social environment, the family members, friends, and communities within which one is raised make an immense difference. Healthcare itself has a certain cluster of virtues that are emphasized and practiced throughout the education and professional development of caregivers at every level of patient care. One of the most important virtues in the history of healthcare professionalism is called altruism. Altruism is the prioritizing of the needs of the other (in this case, the patient) over one's own needs. What the health professions typically profess is the commitment to give priority to care for the patient. In this relational orientation, other values may be subordinated to the importance of the caring for patients' needs. In the past 50 years or so, attention to such relationships has come to be known as "care ethics."

Care ethics

The care ethic demands that the primary concern of religion and the moral life is the relationship among all involved parties. If, for instance, I am pondering whether or not to lie to someone who asks me how I like a new tie or dress, a care ethic, founded upon the caring quality of relationships, would prioritize the depth and details of those relationships over other senses of duty or concern for consequences. To use a more difficult example, if one holds deep moral convictions that abortion should never be allowed and a close friend asks to be accompanied to an abortion clinic for emotional support, a care orientation to religion and spirituality might compel providing such support.

But what is it about the relationships with others that provides such a strong orientation to clinical interactions with patients? Traditionally, relational or caring aspects of patient interactions have been especially associated with nursing. Nurses are the warm, caring professionals while physicians may be regarded more as the ones who do the hard analysis and decision making. In other words, the curing aspects of patient interactions are traditionally associated with physicians (Jecker 2004: 371). With the gradual ascendance of a more relational approach to medical care, this traditional dynamic has been evolving in the direction of a mutually supportive, caregiving team.

One of the central tenets of the care ethic is to emphasize human interdependence as opposed to human independence and individualism. As Nel Noddings puts it in the introduction to the second edition of her seminal work, "Virtually all care theorists make the relational more fundamental than the individual" (Noddings 2013). All individual actions have immense ripple effects in the lives of others in relationship to the person. Recognizing and accounting for this interdependence is essential. The force of personal autonomy is somewhat blunted by this emphasis if autonomy is taken to be atomistic and individualized. And the extent and influence of one's personal moral actions are highlighted in this approach. Again, the point here is not to completely discount other elements important to religion and the moral life, but to prioritize relationships with others. To additionally highlight the narrative approach to religion, a care approach calls for attention to the story of one's life and relationships.

A narrative approach is an important element of a robust concern for others in a relationship-based religious life. For example, if the stories a person or her family have always told about abortion are condemnatory, then the previously mentioned request from a friend to accompany her will make for a particularly difficult decision. On the other hand, if those stories have always sought to extend understanding and grace, there is likely to be a more favorable disposition toward accompanying the friend.

Further, when someone is hospitalized, those of us who care for patients realize our care is extended to that patient's family precisely because of the significant relationships within that family. Those relationships may be functional or dysfunctional, pleasant or unpleasant, but we intuitively recognize this important approach to the manner with which we reach out to the family.

Let this focus on the interdependence of our moral lives launch us into our final concern, namely, how we manage our religion in relation to the religions of those we care for in clinical healthcare. Historically, religion and politics are topics that we all agree not to fight about. In healthcare, particularly in pluralist America, we enter a world where our interactions with others of different faiths challenge us daily. What do we make of this challenge? What are the key areas of religious instruction on ethics and morality that enable us to respect all persons for whom we care?

Religion and spirituality

It is increasingly common in contemporary Western culture to distinguish between religion and spirituality. Religion is typically associated with the belief systems and practices of established faith traditions. Spirituality, in contrast, is typically associated with the personal search for meaning of individuals. Of course, personal spirituality may be linked to a religious tradition. But in many of today's cultures, the linkage between individual spiritual journeys and organized religious traditions has been diminished. For our purposes in this chapter, we note this distinction, but we have chosen to include both religion and spirituality in our discussion of spiritually nurturing and respectful patient care.

Perceptive healthcare professionals often notice their patients' faith or spirituality can be among their most important resources for coping with serious illness or injury. Failure to take these resources into account represents less than optimal care for many patients. On the other hand, spiritual care of patients who may come from many different faith traditions, as well as those who would benefit from spiritual attention but have no identifiable religious commitments, requires following some carefully chosen norms. Here, we discuss five such guides for compassionate care (Winslow and Wehtje-Winslow 2007: 63–66):

1. Understand the patient's religious needs and resources.
2. Follow the expressed wishes of the patient, to the extent this is feasible.
3. Do not prescribe or pressure patients to adopt new practices or convictions.
4. Do not proscribe the patient's religious practices or resources.
5. Understand your own religious convictions, practices, and resources.

Understand the patient's religious needs and resources

Most of us live in highly pluralistic cultures when it comes to religion and spirituality. This means that no single faith tradition or religious vision will have dominance. Given this reality, it is important to permit patients to self-identify whatever they wish to have known about their spiritual needs and resources. Non-intrusive conversations that welcome such exploration are best facilitated in a context that carefully avoids stereotyping based on a patient's apparent ethnicity or perceived cultural heritage. People differ. And even within a named faith tradition, there may be a wide range of personal beliefs and practices. All of the major religions have numerous, distinctive iterations of their faith. We suggest finding thoughtful ways to welcome patients' expression of their own spiritual journey and its significance at this point in their lives. We offer the following script as one example of a way to open such a conversation: "Faith is often important to people when they need healthcare. Is there anything you want us to know about your faith or spiritual practices that might be helpful in your care?"

The hope is to open a pathway of discovery with the patient. No particular script will be suitable for all occasions, patients, or caregivers. A better method is for the caregiver to develop an approach with which he or she feels confident. The goal of such conversations is to help the patient identify her or his own religious or spiritual resources and then permit the patient to express to caregivers how these resources may be helpful in planning for the best possible care. The purpose of these conversations should not be an attempt to bring about a patient's conversion to a new religious tradition.

Follow the expressed wishes of the patient, to the extent this is feasible

As noted earlier, it is often difficult to find the best balance among the principles of respecting the patient's autonomy, providing significant health benefits, and avoiding harm to the patient. Traditionally, the practice of medicine has been shaped by the expectation of paternalism, or the belief that the important decisions about the patient's care should be made unilaterally by the healthcare professionals, especially the physician in charge. After all, it was the physician who was expected to have the greatest knowledge of the science and art of medical care. So whose judgment should govern when caregivers perceive that the patient's beliefs, decisions, and practices may be harmful to his or her health? This question may be peculiarly perplexing when the patient, influenced by strongly held religious beliefs, makes decisions that seem inimical to the usual goals of healthcare. Those goals were usually informed by clinical considerations that had little, if anything, to do with the patient's religious convictions. Learning to navigate the caregiving territory that includes clinical goals of the healthcare team, the personal spiritual goals of the patient, and the established norms of society requires artfulness, creativity, and balance. In finding the balance, it is the settled ethical conviction of our society that we begin with the competent patient's expressed wishes.

The priority our culture gives to patient autonomy is tempered, however, by the professional responsibilities of healthcare providers to offer only those reasonable treatment alternatives for which there is adequate scientific evidence. Healthcare professions are never required to offer or to provide treatment alternatives that, in their professional judgment, are unwarranted in light of scientific evidence. It is imperative for caregivers to maintain personal integrity within the boundaries of their professional knowledge and ethical commitments. If the values of caregivers and care recipients clash, honest attempts to preserve the personal integrity of all those involved can help to reduce moral distress. Such distress may arise from a dissonance of values in a variety of healthcare settings. Specifically, religious convictions sometimes do generate conflicts associated with relatively high levels of distress. Occasionally, such distress may be ameliorated by the caregiver's reassignment to care for other patients with whom there is no dissonance. Healthcare organizations have a wide range of policies that govern the degree to which conscientious objection is allowed as an acceptable option for caregivers. Such policies, in our experience, are rarely invoked. But when needed, they can provide a useful means to manage distress and conflict. Making provision for the conscientious convictions of all members of the healthcare team is one way to ensure that persons of integrity can serve.

Within this context of the balance of caring for one's self and for one's patients, a further word about altruism is in order. Altruism is the purposeful placement of the needs of another person over one's own needs. Altruistic acts tend to flow from the actor's sense of compassion in relationship to the needs of others. Every major religion described in this book espouses the virtue of compassionate altruism. Today's healthcare would benefit from careful reflection on the importance of this virtue. This is especially true in cultures that valorize self-gratifying actions, and less often highlight the essential value of altruism. One ethical implication of a commitment to serve altruistically is the willingness to accommodate the religious needs and respect the religious resources of patients and their families, even when this creates some discomfort for caregivers. A further implication is that caring for inpatients should never include prescribing the adoption of new religious practices or convictions.

Do not prescribe or pressure patients to adopt new practices or convictions

Caregivers interact with patients in a wide variety of settings, some of which may be conducive to conversations about religion, faith, spirituality, and personal practices. As a general rule, however, restraint should be exercised when it comes to introducing religious ideas that are foreign to the patients and their families. This is all the more important as the critical nature of the patient's illness becomes more acute. Despite occasional stories of deathbed religious conversions, seeking to proselytize is ethically inappropriate and disrespectful in the clinical setting. Even though some religious caregivers may be passionate about witnessing for their faith and desirous of helping patients share in that faith, such passion needs to be tempered by the fact that patients are vulnerable. In a religiously pluralistic culture, healthcare is not the proper setting for seeking religious converts.

Of course, it can happen that a patient will request information and insight from a religiously devout caregiver. Even so, an abundance of caution is in order because of patients' vulnerability when they are in critical need of care. The caregiving context usually includes family members and friends of the patient. So, conversations about faith are often not limited to the individual patient. Whole-person care requires paying attention to the patient's social and familial realities. The insights of narrative ethics and care ethics, as mentioned earlier in this chapter, can be enlightening in this regard. They may make caregivers more aware of the stories within which the patients live their lives, including the final chapters of those lives. The key insights of narrative and care ethics may also enliven healthcare professionals' willingness to respect the personal relationships that affect patients' lives.

Do not proscribe the patient's religious practices or resources

This is the complementary norm to that of forswearing the prescription of new religious practices and beliefs. Today's healthcare, governed as it is by many state and federal requirements, is highly controlled and monitored. Many healthcare facilities must forbid certain practices related to religion as it may be practiced in patients' homes or faith communities. For instance, the burning of candles is prohibited for safety reasons. Many hospitals have a "no fragrance" policy that forbids caregivers and families from engaging in the use of any essential oils or incense, thus ruling out some religious rituals as they are customarily practiced. This point came to the fore in a recent case involving one of the authors (Carr). A Hmong family's shaman came to the hospital to help care for a child. Though open to allowing for such involvement, the hospital had to forbid any ritual that entailed burning or smoke.

Additionally, though not necessarily related to religious practice, something as simple as bringing flowers to patients may be forbidden. Herbal products that some may use in the belief that they enhance health will normally need scrutiny by the hospital's pharmacists. Such natural remedies will likely need to be brought to the pharmacy in original packaging for inspection and approval before being allowed into use by the patient. Drug interactions with natural remedies are a relatively new and critical matter requiring caution as Western medicine and non-Western medicine come into the pluralistic mix of modern healthcare in America.

Understand your own religious convictions, practices, and resources

The human character trait of self-reflection is present in each of us at varying levels. Any person who can meaningfully say the words, "I said to myself," must understand that the "I" who is the agent can subject the "Me" to examination. Some of us practice this virtue more easily than others. The role of self-reflection is essential in clinical healthcare professionals. All professionals may benefit from enhanced self-reflection. But what is nice for all professions can be a critical necessity for those professionals who care for patients in hospitals if the goal is genuine and effective whole-person care.

In common parlance, knowing oneself is essential to being open to knowing another person. By knowing oneself we mean to emphasize the fact that exploration and expansion of our knowledge of the world's religions necessarily expands our sense of self. We cannot fully understand what others believe within a vacuum. When we learn what others believe we necessarily compare and contrast what we ourselves believe. This comparison and contrasting process can take a number of default perspectives. For instance, a person might say to her or himself, "nothing I might learn about another religion will ever affect the things I currently believe." Alternatively, a person might be so open to the beliefs of another such that nothing of one's present beliefs will remain intact – everything might be changed by exposure and subsequent adoption of the beliefs of the other. Historically, a well-established function in religious studies was that of apologetics and polemics. An apologist for a particular religious tradition takes every opportunity to defend the rightness of his or her faith while often attempting to demonstrate its superiority over the faith of others. Through polemical arguments, the religious beliefs and practices of other traditions are thus rejected and characterized as false and perhaps even demonic.

In our view, healthcare professionals may positively benefit from deep and abiding religious and spiritual convictions and practices, but they must refrain from engaging in apologetics or polemics in the clinical care of patients. Respectful relationships with patients and with caregiving colleagues require that such potentially contentious approaches to religion or spirituality be set aside. Honesty about one's own convictions and a willingness to exercise humility in sharing them are essential to the ethical, compassionate practice of healthcare professionals.

Bibliography

Beauchamp, T., and Childress, J. (2019) *Principles of Biomedical Ethics*, 8th ed. New York: Oxford University Press.

Borba, M. (2002) *Building Moral Intelligence: The Seven Essential Virtues That Teach Kids to Do the Right Thing*. San Francisco: Jossey-Bass: A Wiley Imprint.

Hauerwas, S., and Jones, LG., eds (1989) *Why Narrative: Readings in Narrative Theology*. Grand Rapids: Eerdmans.

Herdt, JA. (2008) *Putting on Virtue: The Legacy of the Splendid Vices*. Chicago: University of Chicago Press.

Hunter, KM. (2004) "Narrative," *Encyclopedia of Bioethics*. San Francisco: Macmillan Reference USA, Thompson Gale.

Jecker, N. (2004) "Care: Contemporary Ethics of Care," *Encyclopedia of Bioethics*, San Francisco: Macmillan Reference USA, Thompson Gale.

Jonsen, AR. (1991) "Of Balloons and Bicycles – Or – the Relationship Between Ethical Theory and Practical Judgment," *Hastings Center Report*, 21(5): 14–16.

Jonsen, AR., Siegler, M., and Winslade, W. (2021) *Clinical Ethics: A Practical Approach to Ethical Decision Making in Clinical Medicine*, 9th ed. New York: McGraw-Hill.

Nelson, HL. (1997) *Stories and Their Limits: Narrative Approaches to Bioethics*. New York: Routledge.

Noddings, N. (2013) *Caring: A Relational Approach to Ethics and Moral Education*. Los Angeles: University of California Press.

Pellegrino, E., and Thomasma, D. (1993) *The Virtues in Medical Practice*. New York: Oxford University Press.

Rawls, J. (1971) *A Theory of Justice*. Cambridge: Belknap of Harvard University Press.

Sommers, C., and Sommers, F. (2004) *Vice & Virtue in Everyday Life: Introductory Readings in Ethics*, 6th ed.. Belmont, CA: Wadsworth/Thompson Learning.

Winslow, G., and Wehtje-Winslow, B. (2007) "Ethical Boundaries of Spiritual Care," *Medical Journal of Australia*, 186(10): S63–S66.

3 Religion and public health

Andy Lampkin and Mark F. Carr

Introduction

Humans are religious. In every epoch of recorded history, we find religion at the center of human life and wellbeing. In private life and the public square, religious traditions play a significant role in the lives of people all around the world. Estimates say that more than 80% of the world's population identify with a religion (Global Religious Landscape 2012). Thomas A. Tweed, in *Religion: A Very Short Introduction*, argues that religion "is simultaneously bringing people together and pulling people apart" such that those of us engaged in the public space of healthcare should "understand religion." "It does not matter if you find religion compelling" or not. What matters, according to Tweed, "is that billions around the world practice a faith—and that they act from it" (Tweed 2020: xi).

In this brief chapter we attempt to capture the essence of the effect of religion on the public's health. How does a community, society, or nation orient its shared life around health and wellbeing? As we explore this topic, we do not need to argue that religion is essential to public wellbeing, neither do we wish to hide from the ugly realities of the illicit use of powerful religions on private and public life. Our simple assertion is that we must explicitly attend to religion in our lives so as to optimize the public's health. We explore this thesis in three parts: first, Religion and health; second, Public and the public's health; and third, Religion and public health. We finish with a note on the challenges facing religion and public health in the United States.

Religion and health

Thirty plus years of research illustrates a close association between religion and health. Professionals at major medical centers have incorporated religious and spiritual content as part of the care of patients. Health science education has been exploring the role of religion in the medical curriculum. There is sustained interest in religion and health and a recognition of the significant role religion and spirituality play in the lives of individuals.

There is a tremendous amount of literature produced on the subject matter. What has come into focus is that religion plays a significant role in the lives of individuals for their health and wellbeing. When it comes to health outcomes there is wide-spread agreement that religion affects physical and mental health, a sense of wellbeing, lifestyle behaviors, and one's ability to cope with the stresses of life (Chatters 2000).

DOI: 10.4324/9781003288862-3

Within these broad conceptual categories there are explanations for what may be going on. For example, within the category of physical health outcomes, it is theorized that religion is instrumental in shaping behaviors. Religions prescribe and proscribe behaviors that are acceptable and unacceptable that in turn have health consequences.

There is a positive association between religious involvement and social support. Belonging to a religious community provides members with social ties and social reciprocity. In addition, religious practices such as prayer and communion engender a connection with others. Religious beliefs, through teachings and worship practices, may encourage a positive attitude and outlook on life, a sense of self-worth, and positive self-esteem (Chatters 2000).

Although the research has shown many positive connections between religion and health, the association is mixed. There are also negative aspects of religious involvement. There can be religious teachings that are inconsistent with scientific knowledge. Such teaching may discourage the use of modern medicine. Negative aspects of religion can be related to difficult or problematic relationships within the community. Religion as a social support network carries with it enormous amounts of social pressure and when one is on the wrong side of religious norms, one can experience stress and anxiety.

Religious practices and public health

Researchers recognized the role of religion on public health. It is theorized that religion functions as social support, social control, and a source of social capital (Idler 2014; Shapiro 2021). We have already discussed social control and social support. Through social capital, religion directly impacts population health. Religious communities produce and manage social institutions such as schools, health clinics, hospitals, grass roots organizations, and social services entities. These institutions and network of social services very often impact public health.

Moreover, religion through complex beliefs, rituals, and practices shapes how we experience and impact the world. These rituals are often framed around frequency – daily, weekly, annual, and one-time practices. These ritualized practices may have consequences for individual wellbeing and public health.

Daily religious practices

For Christians and Muslims, for instance, daily prayer is an important spiritual discipline. Prayer allows individuals to connect with something outside of themselves – God. Muslims pray five times a day facing the east, in the direction of Mecca, Saudi Arabia, where the holy Kaaba centers the attention of the faithful. Meditation, a similar practice as prayer, is essential to many eastern religions including Buddhism. For Buddhists who practice meditation it effects levels of depression, diabetes control, addiction control, and suicide risk (Negi & Ozawa-de Silva 2014; Chatters 2000). The practices of prayer and meditation are known to reduce stress and the body's inflammation response, control anxiety, and promote emotional health, and may reduce age-related memory loss, improve sleep, help treat addictions, help control pain, and decrease blood pressure.

The daily ritualized dietary practices of avoiding some foods and consuming others have been shown to have significant health consequences. Vegetarianism among

Seventh-day Adventists has been documented to have positive health consequences (Grant & Montenegro 2014). Tai-chi in Taoism improves balance, prevents falls, reduces musculoskeletal pain, and improves overall quality of life (Reinders 2014).

Weekly religious practices

Attendance at the Synagogue, Mosque, and Church routinely shows positive health effects in research. Attendance at faith community gatherings is a source of social support and social connection through networks. It has been suggested that a "good social network can have more health benefits than giving up smoking" (Launay 2015). The sense of being socially connected is important for one's sense of wellbeing.

In religious communities where singing and/or chanting is common, research shows positive health benefits. One Oxford study concluded that choir singing improves health and happiness (Launay 2015). The therapeutic effect of music, singing, and chanting creates a sense of wellbeing, relives stress, exercises the brain, stimulates the immune response, improves breathing, improves posture and muscle tension, reduces pain, and eases the effects of dementia (Launay 2015; Saliers 2014; Wan et al. 2010).

Annual religious practices

Many religions have annual celebrations. Hindus annually celebrate Krishna Janmashtami, Muslims celebrate Ramadan, adherents of Judaism celebrate Yom Kippur. These yearly events usually include some form of ritual fasting. Fasting has a wide range of health benefits from improving cognitive performance, reducing inflammation, improving blood sugar control, and increasing physical endurance (An-Na'im 2014; Link 2022). Researchers have also discovered the positive effects of fasting on chronic kidney disease, fertility-related issues, tear secretion, sleep patterns, cholesterol, stroke, frequency of migraines, heart health, blood pressure, cholesterol levels, and the prevention of neurodegenerative disorders.

One-time religious practices

Some of the one-time religious rituals illustrate the occasionally negative realities of religious practices. Female Genital Mutilation/Cutting (FGMC) as a puberty rite, for instance, is known to cause a host of female health-related problems. The American *Centers for Disease Control and Prevention (CDC)*, citing the *World Health Organization*, defines FGMC as "all procedures involving partial or total removal of the external female genitalia or other injury to the female genital organs for non-medical reasons" (CDC 2020). According to the CDC more than 200 million girls and women have experienced FGMC worldwide. FGMC is integral to multiple religions and cultures and the lines of demarcation are hard to draw. Nonetheless, FGMC has no positive health benefits.

Perhaps oddly, the typically one-time practice of baptism by immersion often has negative public health consequences. When baptism happens in polluted bodies of water, adherents are subjected to waterborne diseases. Fred De Sam Lazaro, in a PBS special, brought attention to the Christian practice of baptism in the dangerously polluted parts of the Jordan River (Lazaro 2010). This is not only an issue in Jerusalem but in many other parts of the world including South Africa and some Latin American countries.

Religious ritual after death can also have negative public health consequences. Death practices vary among religious traditions. Hindus in India, for instance, conduct ritual cremation of their beloved deceased on the banks of rivers. The holiest place for these cremation ceremonies is in the city of Benares, India, on the banks of the Ganges River.

Hindus believe that these rites free the soul from the cycle of death and rebirth and are necessary for salvation. But a *Washington Post* newspaper article revealed the negative effects on the environment when tens of thousands of the dead are cremated daily in the same place. In the article, *India's Burial Rites Put Nature at Risk*, journalists noted that 20,000 cremations per day results in a river clogged with human ashes (George 2003). Not to mention the consumption of firewood and resultant atmospheric smoke. Each cremation requires roughly 650 pounds of wood to burn the body prompting intense environmental concerns. The article notes that "the ashes of millions of dead have turned the water into a stinking, polluted swirl. Worse, since wood is expensive, bodies sometimes are thrown into the river half-burned" (George 2003).

The final disposition of the dead is a scared responsibility of family members in most religions. These practices, while honoring their dead, may create public health crises. In parts of the world where infectious diseases are a common cause of sickness and death, how one cares for the dying, handles the body, and later disposes of it may have public health consequences.

Religious rituals matter to public health. To be clear, it's not the practice of cremation or baptism by immersion that is problematic. It is that these rituals are performed in contexts and environmental settings that are not safe or create unsafe conditions that should raise our moral concern.

Public and the public's health

Although defining public health is occasionally contested, the *American Public Health Association* (APHA) defines it as the promotion and protection of "the health of people and the communities where they live, learn, work and play" (APHA 2022b). Clearly, this is an expansive effort that includes many disciplines and coordination among them. Social workers and nutritionists, first responders and school nurses, epidemiologists and government health officials, bench sciences, social sciences, community and behavioral health, law, and public policy, all come together to protect and promote our health and wellbeing. Note in the APHA's expanded list of "Essential Public Health Services" areas within which faith communities might play an integral part:

1. Assess and monitor population health.
2. Investigate, diagnose and address health hazards and root causes.
3. Communicate effectively to inform and educate.
4. Strengthen, support and mobilize communities and partnerships.
5. Create, champion and implement policies, plans and laws.
6. Utilize legal and regulatory actions.
7. Enable equitable access.
8. Build a diverse and skilled workforce.
9. Improve and innovate through evaluation, research, and quality improvement.
10. Build and maintain a strong organizational infrastructure for public health.

(APHA 2022b)

Public health is not a static discipline, it's always in the process of becoming, ever changing, bringing to bear the necessary intellectual, human, and technological resources, to address the issues it confronts. Public health looks different depending on the social context and social factors at play. Variables such as country status (developing or developed), industrial or agrarian, regions and contextual factors within countries (urban or rural, coastal, or inland), multicultural or multiethnic are all factors that shape public health work.

Historically, public health has focused on clean drinking water, sanitation, and control of infectious diseases. Contemporary public health includes other concerns and initiatives, such as vaccinations, air quality, handwashing, smoking cessation, obesity education and reduction, access to healthcare, HIV/AIDS prevention, occupational safety, and reproductive health (Rosen 1993; APHA 2022b). Social factors such as adequate housing, safe communities and safe work environments, convenient transportation, access to healthy foods, access to healthcare, and economic development, all influences health and well-being in very significant ways, and hence the public's health.

Conceptual foundation

The conceptual foundation of public health begins with the whole population and moves to the individual. This is an important distinction from the perspective of healthcare and medicine which is founded on the individual patient/provider relationship. The public is the whole, not the individual and not simply a gathering of individuals. Put clearly, the needs of the individual are sometimes necessarily overridden by the needs of the whole. Americans typically approach life from an individualistic perspective, so accounting for the prioritization of the population in public health can be a challenge. Ethical theories that justify the prioritization of the community over the individual, such as Utilitarianism, provide the foundation for many public health practices and priorities. Similarly, local, state, and federal health policies must focus on whole populations while attempting to protect individual privacy and rights. This is not an easy balance.

Public health has always been a strong advocate of using science and the careful data it produces as the foundation for establishing standards of health practice for citizens. One reason we can assume safe drinking water from our taps and safe foods to purchase in our stores is the regulatory standards of our government public health departments. Scientific research and data face many challenges of substance as well as misinformation today. A robust exchange of research method and practice is a welcome part of the scientific ethos and research community.

However, the truths established by epidemiological science remain factual regardless of whether you and I believe it. A pathogen is a pathogen and that does not change with political parties, social ideology, or religious devotion. Public health and its ability to help us create and sustain a healthy community absolutely depends upon acceptance of good science and data. The public health discipline, profession, and role within government must of course be scrutinized in its work. Such scrutiny, however, must be in balance with the good science and public-minded citizenry from the finest expressions of our faith traditions.

What follows this reality, then, is a vigorous effort to gather the information necessary to understand and analyze epidemiological effects and trends. If the public (including persons committed to our faith traditions) is unwilling to be involved and helpful in this process, there is little hope for effective means to fight disease. Capturing and creating useful information and tools is essential for public health officials to do their work well. Returning to one of our earlier points, religious communities in America are indispensable to this effort. Our society must find beneficial ways to communicate and partner with each other to the positive end of health and wellbeing for all.

Principal concerns

One of the most prevalent and consistent problems in public health in America regards the disparate outcomes for marginalized persons and communities. The health and wellbeing of marginalized groups of people is markedly lower than average. The dynamics of this problem revolve around power, position, wealth, and protection of privilege through federal, state, and local law, policy, and practice. These disparities are well researched and known by public health agencies and all levels of public policy makers; they are not debatable. They persist for reasons that are both complex and clear.

Understanding health disparities and health equities

According to Healthy People 2020, a

> health disparity is a particular type of health difference that is closely linked with economic, social, or environmental disadvantage. Health disparities adversely affect groups of people who have systematically experienced greater social or economic obstacles to health based on their racial or ethnic group, religion, socioeconomic status, gender, age or mental health; cognitive, sensory, or physical disability; sexual orientation or gender identity; geographic location; or other characteristics historically linked to discrimination or exclusion.
>
> (Healthy People 2020 n.d.)

This expansive definition communicates the social factors that are implicated in health disparities – access to healthcare, environmental conditions, poverty and other forms of economic insecurity, individual and behavioral factors, and educational inequalities (CDC 2013). By identifying the social contributions to health, this definition embraces the social determinates of health model. It notes the significance of social hierarchy and contingent factors such as gender, sexual orientation, physical and other forms of disabilities, class, racial and ethnic group membership. Overall, it shows us that where one falls within the social hierarchy has a direct relationship to one's health. This definition also takes seriously environmental factors, that where one lives, grows, and works contributes to one's health. Access to safe drinking water, high quality foods, adequate and safe housing, the absence of environmental hazards, and access to healthcare are the environmental conditions that impact human health.

This definition also makes clear that every health difference or disparate health outcome is not necessary a health disparity. A health disparity is a particular type of health difference that is linked to our social arrangements – which can always be altered. Health and health outcomes that are the consequence of natural endowments and are not amenable to changes in social policies and practices are not health disparities. It is beyond the scope of this chapter to fully explore this line of reasoning. For now, it is important to note that natural differences in health status and health outcomes exist between individuals and groups. For instance, the differences in incidences between men and women related to prostate cancer and breast cancer are not examples of health disparities. Though the incidence rates are disparate, they occur naturally and are largely explained by the genetic differences between men and women.

A clear understanding of health disparities is necessary because health disparities are ethically unacceptable. As such, religious communities and public health practitioners have keen interests in ameliorating the health disparities status quo. Equally important is a thorough understanding of health equity. As a social norm, health equity functions as a goal or objective of many public health efforts. Health equity is concerned with the reduction of unwanted health disparities and a "striving for the highest possible standard of health for all people and giving special attention to the needs of those at the greatest risk of poor health, based on social conditions" (Braveman 2014: 2).

The principle of health equity orients our moral attention. It further informs the types of resources and efforts that are required to meet our shared goal of health for all. The principle of health equity is grounded in other social values, international laws, and human rights. These social values, international agreements, and global consensus advance the right to health, and the right to the social resources necessary to be healthy. These rights are applicable to all persons as they are grounded in the principles of nondiscrimination and equality among persons and groups (UNESCO 2005).

Health equity as social justice

It is important to note that health disparities, health equity, and social justice are interwoven concepts. Social justice is what we all are owed. As Braveman notes, "health equity means social justice in health." She explains further, "no one is denied the possibility to be healthy for belonging to a group that has been economically/socially disadvantaged" (Braveman 2014: 3). Health disparities burden many populations of people across a whole range of health conditions including, but not limited to, cancers, chronic kidney disease, chronic pain, dementia, diabetes, heart disease, infectious disease, mental health, oral health, overweight and obesity, respiratory diseases, and sexually transmitted infections (Healthy People 2030 n.d.). These disease conditions disparately impact various populations including racial and ethnic minorities, LGBT+ persons, people with disabilities, immigrants, and children. Health disparities also show up based on geography, levels of educational attainment, and social economic status.

Without offering fully developed arguments around the thesis of health equity as social justice, this chapter offers an argument that health is an important value to individuals across their lifespan. Human beings want to be healthy and live lives void of physical and mental impairments. Moreover, health is necessary for individuals to achieve their life plans and goals. As discussed earlier, health is achieved and maintained by the social conditions in which one lives, grows, and works. It is this grounding that situates health as social justice. Contemporary philosophers such as Amartya Sen, John Rawls, Norman Daniels, Ronald Dworkin, Michael Walzer, and Thomas Pogge have all reflected on health in the realm of social justice. To be sure, any serious discussion about social justice must consider health and wellbeing. Norman Daniels reasoned that health is a human good and of special moral importance (Daniels 2008). He argued that health is the kind of good that is necessary for people to pursue other important goods and ends.

Because of the special importance of health, it is a basic societal entitlement, a key feature of a just society.

Theories and ideas of social justice are helpful as they serve as a guide to our moral concerns and common aspirations to be healthy, avoid disability, and needless suffering. Like philosophers, theologians from every world religion have long argued for human flourishing. Human health is an important value that should be pursued; in some sense flourishing can be seen as a religious duty. Disease, illness, and disability are to be anticipated and may be countered through prayer, ritual, and spiritual disciplines. This kind of theological thinking is what animated religious groups to establish and operate hospitals and clinics. Grounded in the traditions of the world's religions are social duties to care for ourselves and promote the wellbeing of our neighbors.

Thus, it is at the intersection of health disparities, health equity, and social justice that public health practitioners and religious communities can and should engage one another. Both groups have been historically concerned with the promotion of health, reduction of disease, and leveling the playing field by advocating for alterations in social conditions, social policies, and practices that create the disparate health outcomes in the first place.

Thus, the major gaps in life expectancies that exist between highest and lowest incomes that move on a gradient should raise our moral concern. Researchers have been able to map life expectancy between US zip codes and found up to 20 years in disparity based on zip codes in very close proximity (Ducharme & Wolfson 2019; Owens-Young 2020). Racial and ethnic disparities have been discovered to be hiding in plain sight for more than a century across many health outcomes including infant mortality, life expectancies, exposure to environmental pollutant, and maternal mortality (Radley et al. 2021). These disparities fall outside our societal norms of justice and stand in need of correction. Health equity is a principal concern in today's public health work. Our task is to find the root causes for these unjust disparities and correct them with substantive practice and policy adjustments.

Two widely respected sources of the information on healthcare inequities are:

- *The United States Centers for Disease Control and Prevention Social Vulnerability Index* (ATSDR, 2022)
- *The Area Deprivation Index* (Center for Health Disparities Research, n.d.)

Implications regarding religion and public health

Our obligation to our neighbors, understood as a universal principle of human behavior, is at the root of building a more trusting relationship between religion and public health. It is rare in the history of the world's religions for specific faith traditions to focus on the commonalities of our shared life. Characteristically we hear all the distinct reasons why this or that religion is the best. We are routinely shown how bad others are while being shown how lovely our own religion/faith is. It is the distinctive features of a religion that are thought to be so special. When this attitude of comparison and denigration of the other becomes the prevailing posture within the public square we all suffer.

Furthermore, when this same distrustful and polemical disposition exists between faith communities and the government agencies that attend to the public's health, we all suffer. Unless you were asleep through the COVID-19 pandemic you have seen and experienced such animosity and distrust among us. We reject this destructive pattern and urge all parties to refocus on the commonalities among us, on the common good for our societies.

Religion and public health: contested spaces

Tension of public and private interest.

There are numerous examples of public health practitioners successfully working closely with faith community leaders. Religious communities are prime sites for public health partnership. Partnership and cooperation are things that many faith communities are willing to do with public health. However, the public health community and the faith community may not share the same values even when they may have a common goal. They are often animated by very different understandings of the world.

Declarations of religious freedom, for instance, can place public health and religious communities at odds. Many in the anti-vaccination faction make claims to religious liberty to support their position against vaccination requirements for public school attendance. In April 2021, a lawsuit was filed against Connecticut State Department of Education, by three mothers representing three different faith traditions, Christianity (Catholic), Islam (Muslim), and Greek Orthodox faith (Christian). In the case, *We the Patriots USA, INC vs. Connecticut Office of Early Childhood Development*, these mothers objected to the repeal of a Connecticut law that provided for a religious exemption for vaccination for children to attend public or private schools (*We the Patriots...* 2022).

The new law did not allow a religious exemption for children who did not already have a religious exemption. The parents claimed they had a religious right to reject vaccinations and their children should be allowed to attend schools unvaccinated. This of course would put at risk children, who are unable to be vaccinated for health reasons, in danger. This highlights a tension between individual rights and the common good, and contested space between religion and public health. We know that vaccines are safe and effective. However, individuals should enjoy religious liberty and protections from unwanted intrusion into personal health choices. This tension is not easily resolved since the common good must, at times, override individual choice.

To be sure, religious communities do not exist to serve public health ends. Religious contribution to public health may be more serendipitous even though they naturally and organically flow from religious beliefs. Public health practitioners need to be sensitive to the many possible conflicts that could ruin relationships with religious groups. Moreover, public health practitioners must resist the temptation to oversimplify the meaning of religious values, teachings, and practices. Religious beliefs cannot be reduced to discrete health behaviors. Such an approach would completely misunderstand, fail to appreciate, and disrespect the role that religion plays in health, and overall wellbeing of individuals and communities.

Challenges facing religion and public health

We recognize the difficulty of seeking commonality among the world's religions. Pushing toward establishing and enhancing existing open and trustful communication between public health and our religious communities is obviously challenging. Nonetheless, we are compelled toward the common good in the interface of religion and public health. We must become better partners for our overall wellbeing. Public health officials and faith community leaders must avoid opposition and seek cooperation.

As an ethical mandate, public health practitioners must appreciate religion on its own terms as a quest for God and/or a search for meaning in a highly complex world full of existential challenges. Religion is a conceptual meaning-making system that informs behaviors that impact health and wellbeing. Faith communities have served in the past and will continue in the future to act as social agents that promote health and communal wellbeing. The public health community must seek to understand religious motivations and framing on their own terms if they are to be successful in working with faith communities. Thus, one ethical challenge is to avoid reducing faith practices to health behaviors. As Idler eloquently notes, "seeing faith-based intervention as no different than interventions in the secular realm is mistaken ..." (Idler 2014: 409).

A second ethical challenge to avoid is the exclusion of religion and religious communities as an important social determinant of health and a resource in public health practice. This is an important moral concern. Religious communities concerned with and committed to individual and communal wellbeing are an essential resource for public health practice considering that 80% of the world populations identify with some religion.

A third ethical challenge is that public health ethics is its own field of inquiry, with a set of concerns, approach to ethics, and what counts as ethical engagement with the public. In the U.S. context public health ethics has established itself as distinct and different from medical ethics or clinical ethics. As public health is grounded on social concerns, it operates on core ethical values such as professionalism and trust, health justice and equity, health and safety, interdependence and solidarity, human rights and civil liberties, and inclusivity and engagement (APHA 2022a). These values are good and may be universally applicable. The ethical challenge, however, is to actively demonstrate that the ethical values of the public health profession are indeed complimentary and commensurate with our religious communities. Public health practitioners must demonstrate through ethical practices public health core values as they work with religious communities.

Fourth, as an ethical value, public health professionals must commit to practice the view that no one can be reduced to their religion. Religion is always operating in a complex web of culture, ethnicity, nationality, gender, class, socio-economic status, and an individual's own desires and unique needs. Individuals can transcend the various contingencies of their life. As an ethical mandate they must always be treated as such.

Conclusion

In rather brief form, we have laid out what we take to be an essential posture of faith traditions working with public health officials in our local, regional, and national communities. All parties involved seek the wellbeing of our beloved communities.

Religiously devoted members of our communities are deeply influenced by ideas of wellbeing in their faith traditions. Even among those only nominally committed, habits and lifestyle patterns from their religion regularly influence their behavior. Similarly, public health officials are influenced and monitored in accord with the profession and practice of their discipline. In the public space that we all inhabit it behooves us to do all we can to work together so that all of us, and especially those among us who have suffered disparate healthcare access and outcomes, can enjoy wellbeing. All of us are benefitted by caring for those who have been marginalized. We urge the readers of this text to consider how the embrace of their vocational/professional life can accomplish the goal of widespread wellbeing.

Bibliography

Agency for Toxic Substances and Disease Registry (ATSDR) (2022) "Social Vulnerability Index," Centers for Disease Control and Prevention. www.atsdr.cdc.gov/placeandhealth/svi/at-a-glance_svi.html

American Public Health Association (APHA) (2022a) "Public Health Code of Ethics." www.apha.org/-/media/files/pdf/membergroups/ethics/code_of_ethics.ashx

American Public Health Association (APHA) (2022b) "What is Public Health." www.apha.org/What-is-Public-Health

An-Na'im, A. (2014) "Fasting in Islam," in Idler, EL. (ed.), *Religion as a Social Determinant of Public Health* (pp. 49–56). New York, NY: Oxford University Press.

Braveman P. (2014) "What Are Health Disparities and Health Equity? We Need to Be Clear," *Public health reports (Washington, D.C.: 1974)*, 129(2): 5–8. https://doi.org/10.1177/00333354 9141291S203

Centers for Disease Control (CDC) (2013) "Health Disparities and Inequalities Report 2013." www.cdc.gov/mmwr/pdf/other/su6203.pdf

Centers for Disease Control (CDC) (2020) "Female Genital Mutilation/Cutting (FGMC)." www.cdc.gov/reproductivehealth/womensrh/female-genital-mutilation.html

Center for Health Disparities Research (n.d.) *Neighborhood Atlas*. University of Wisconsin, School of Medicine and Public Health. www.neighborhoodatlas.medicine.wisc.edu

Chatters, LA. (2000) "Religion and Health: Public Health Research and Practice," *Annual Review Public Health*, 21: 335–367. www.annualreviews.org/doi/10.1146/annurev.publhealth.21.1.335

Daniels, N. (2008) *Just Health: Meeting Health Needs Fairly*. New York, NY: Cambridge University Press.

Ducharme, J., and Wolfson, E. (2019) "Your Zip Code Might Determine How Long You Live— and the Difference Could be Decades." *Time*. https://time.com/5608268/zip-code-health/

George, N. (2003) "India's Burial Rites Put Nature at Risk." *The Washington Post*. www.washingtonpost.com/archive/politics/2003/08/17/indias-burial-rites-put-nature-at-risk/404ee316-5ec5-4e28-849a-4adf512a852e/

Grant, H., and Montenegro, J. (2014) "Vegetarianism in Seventh-day Adventism," in Idler, EL. (ed.), *Religion as a Social Determinant of Public Health* (pp. 49–56). New York, NY: Oxford University Press.

Healthy People 2020 (n.d.). https://wayback.archive-it.org/5774/20190703185522/https://www.healthypeople.gov/2020/default

Healthy People 2030 (n.d.). https://health.gov/healthypeople

Idler, EL. (ed.) (2014) "Religion: The Invisible Social Determinant," in Idler, EL. (ed.) *Religion as a Social Determinant of Public Health* (pp. 1–24). New York, NY: Oxford University Press.

Launay, J. (2015) "Choir Singing Improves Health, Happiness – and is the Perfect Ice Breaker." www.ox.ac.uk/research/choir-singing-improves-health-happiness-%E2%80%93-and-perfect-ice breaker

Lazaro, FDS. (2010) "Jordan River Baptism." *Public Broadcasting System, Religion and Ethics Newsweekly*. www.pbs.org/wnet/religionandethics/2010/10/08/october-8-2010-jordan-river-baptisms/7179/

Link, R. (2022) "8 Health Benefits of Fasting, Backed by Science." *Nutrition*, November 21, 2022. www.healthline.com/nutrition/fasting-benefits

Negi, GLT., and Ozawa-de Silva, B. (2014) "Refuge Meditation in Contemporary Buddhism," in Idler, EL. (ed.), *Religion as a Social Determinant of Public Health* (pp. 31–37). New York, NY: Oxford University Press.

Owens-Young, J. (2020) "Zip Code Effect: Neighborhood Can Affect Life Expectancy by 30 Years." *Blue Zones.* www.bluezones.com/2020/02/zip-code-effect-your-neighborhood-determi nes-your-lifespan/

Pew Research Center (2012) "Global Religious Landscape." www.pewresearch.org/religion/2012/ 12/18/global-religious-landscape-exec/

Radley, CD., Baumgartner, JC., Collins, RS., Zephyrin, L., and Schneider, EC. (2021) "Achieving Racial and Ethnic Equity in U.S. Health Care." *The Commonwealth Fund.* www.commonwea lthfund.org/publications/scorecard/2021/nov/achieving-racial-ethnic-equity-us-health-care-state-performance

Reinders, E. (2014) "Taiji (*T'ai-chi*) in Taoism," in Idler, EL. (ed.), *Religion as a Social Determinant of Public Health* (pp. 38–43). New York, NY: Oxford University Press.

Rosen, G. (1993) *A History of Public Health.* Baltimore, Maryland: The Johns Hopkins University Press.

Saliers, D. (2014) "Congregational Hymn Singing in Mainline Protestantism," in Idler, EL. (ed.), *Religion as a Social Determinant of Public Health* (pp. 63–67). New York, NY: Oxford University Press.

Shapiro, E. (2021) "A Protective Canopy: Religious and Social Capital as Elements of a Theory of Religion and Health," *Journal of Religion and Health*, 61: 4466–4480. https://link.springer.com/ article/10.1007/s10943-021-01207-8

Tweed, TA. (2020) *Religion: A Very Short Introduction.* New York, NY: Oxford University Press.

United Nations Educational, Scientific and Cultural Organization (UNESC) (2005) "Universal Declaration on Bioethics and Human Rights." https://en.unesco.org/themes/ethics-science-and-technology/bioethics-and-human-rights

Wan, YC., Ruber, T., Hohmann, A., and Schlaug, G., (2010) "The Therapeutic Effects of Singing in Neurological Disorders," *Music Percepts*, April 1; 27(4): 287–295. www.ncbi.nlm.nih.gov/ pmc/articles/PMC2996848/

We the Patriots U.S., Inc. v. Conn. Office of Early Childhood Development. (2022) Casetext. https://casetext.com/case/we-the-patriots-us-inc-v-conn-office-of-early-childhood-dev

Wolpe, PR., Burnett, W., and Idler, E. (2014) "Religion's Role as a Social Determinant of Twenty-First Century Health: Perspective from the Disciplines," in Idler, EL. (ed.), *Religion as a Social Determinant of Public Health* (pp. 408–419). New York, NY: Oxford University Press.

4 American Indian religions

Carla Gober Park and Roy Kim[1]

Great Spirit Prayer
Oh, Great Spirit, Whose voice I hear in the winds,
And whose breath gives life to all the world,
Hear me, I am small and weak, I need your strength and wisdom.
Let me walk in beauty and make my eyes ever behold the red and purple sunset.
Make my hands respect the things you have made and my ears sharp to hear your voice.
Make me wise so that I may understand the things you have taught my people.
Let me learn the lessons you have hidden in every leaf and rock.
I seek strength, not to be greater than my brother, but to fight my greatest enemy – myself.
Make me always ready to come to you with clean hands and straight eyes.
So when life fades, as the fading sunset, my Spirit may come to you without shame.

(Lakota Sioux Chief Yellow Lark 1887)

Introduction

"You can come in now." The nurse encourages me into the room where my father is having basal cell skin cancer removed from his face. I am unprepared for the sight. There is a hole the size of a quarter in my father's nose where the physician has removed tissue. My father talks and jokes with me, seemingly unaware of the gaping hole. I feel queasy and excuse myself.

My mother joins me in the hall and states the facts simply. "The doctor is examining the tissue to see if he needs to remove more."

More? My mind races back and forth over the events that have brought us here. My father identifies himself as American Indian, of the Cherokee tribe. American Indian artwork lines the walls of one room in his home and he operates in the world with a spirituality and connectedness to all things, including animals and nature. He believes in "natural remedies." Up until the surgery, he wanted to treat the growing mysterious skin changes on his nose with herbs boiled into a thick paste. He applied the herb poultices to his face and later recounted stories of how the poultices "pulled out" the cancer. In one case, he froze the tissue that had been pulled out and used the frozen sample to illustrate his stories. He believed that his "cancer cream" only affected cancer cells, leaving normal skin unaffected. Over time the rest of us watched as the mysterious redness grew larger. Several times we pleaded with him to see a physician. Reluctantly, he consented.

My mother interrupts my thoughts. "The physician says that if we had waited much longer, it might have gone into his brain." As I walk back into the room, her comment

DOI: 10.4324/9781003288862-4

helps me deal with my guilt that I am somehow responsible for his current disfigurement. For the next two months, my dad looks as if he has had a stroke. His mouth is asymmetrical due to nerve disruption. At one point, my father states that if he had to do it over, he would not go to the physician. He believes that God provided natural remedies for every kind of illness and that the herb poultices would have worked if just given time.

Eventually, the wound heals, the nerve returns to normal function and my father's skin looks perfect again, without asymmetry. But his mind is not changed. If the skin cancer returns, he will use the herb remedies. Soon after hearing of his decision, I happen upon an advertisement for a new basal cell skin cancer cream, derived of herbs. It affects only cancer cells, leaving normal skin unaffected.

I am stunned. Was my father correct? Was his concoction similar to the new medical cream in the advertisement? Was I wrong to insist that he get help from a physician? Does the positive outcome justify my insistence? My father did not see Western medicine as "the remedy." For him it was only one of several paths to healing, and not the most important one. Unlike my father, I saw Western medicine as the most important path to healing. We were "dancing between two worlds" (Gustafson 1997).

My father does not represent every indigenous person. He represents the complexities of those who identify as American Indian and of the deep connections between spirituality, nature, and healing. He also represents those whose worlds are not understood. My father and I were dancing between two worlds, as are any two groups who view the world differently. But this dance between Western medicine and that practiced by Native Americans represents more than a negotiation between two belief systems; it represents two ways of knowing and thinking that are affected by histories, ecologies, narratives, and dynamics of power. For David Abram (2010), the body itself is a kind of place, a terrain that can be settled or colonized by others. "Colonization isn't simply the physical occupation of land. It is a process, an operation of power in which one cosmology is extinguished and replaced with another" (Marya & Patel 2021). To be in this dance and to avoid the over-reach of power, one has to be in community, where all involved are perceived as people, rather than objects or noise. Only then does the dance move all involved beyond perceptions of opposition and imbalance of power to a potentially creative space that enlarges the view of the world for all involved and is akin to storytelling itself.

In healthcare clinics across North America, American Indians who enter the clinical world of "Western" medicine enter into this dance. As healthcare providers your ability to both understand and enter into this "dance" will enhance the healing enterprise in your clinic.

Demographics

The United States Census Bureau estimates that as of 2020 there are approximately 7.1 million people in the United States who identify themselves as American Indian or Alaska Native (alone or in combination with other races), amounting to 2.1 percent of the total population. This estimate is projected to go up to 10.1 million within the next 40 years and partially reflects the increasing numbers of people who identify themselves as American Indian (US Census Bureau 2021).

The definition of "Indian" is complex. Many people, including the American Indians themselves, use the terms *American Indian* and *Native American* interchangeably, thus the terms are used interchangeably in this chapter. There is no general consensus on which term is best; however, many desire to be referred to according to the tribal group in which they belong. There are 574 federally recognized tribes and nations in the United States (National Congress of American Indians 2020). The largest American Indian tribes are: Cherokee, Navajo, Choctaw, Chippewa, Sioux, Apache, Blackfeet, Creek (Muscogee), Iroquois, and Lumbee (Centeno 2021). The main Alaska Native tribal groups are: Athabaskan, Tlingit, Haida, and Tsimshian (Alaskan Natives n.d.). These tribes speak over 175 indigenous languages (Acutrans 2020). This only begins to illustrate the diversity within the American Indian and Alaska Native groups. Thus, it is impossible to avoid generalizations that gloss over tribal differences. However, in general, a broader overview is important for basic knowledge.

Further complicating this is that not everyone who identifies as American Indian is actually counted as American Indian. General guidelines have been developed to determine eligibility for health services. By some guidelines, an American Indian is a person who has two qualifications: (1) ancestors living in America before its discovery, and (2) being recognized as American Indian by his or her tribe or community (Cohen 1982). Using this protocol, my father would not be considered an indigenous person, even though both parents are from American Indian descent. He is not currently recognized as American Indian by his tribe, simply because he has not initiated that recognition; however, *he identifies himself* as American Indian.

Today, 60 percent of Native Americans identify as Christians, 35 percent are unaffiliated or unknown, and the remaining are Jewish or "other world religions" (Public Religion Research Institute 2021). Demographics within Native American religion are complex. First, many Native Americans do not regard their spiritual beliefs as religion. There is no word for *religion* in the Native languages. Their religion is a way of life that integrates all aspects of life into a whole, and it is understood entirely within the context of the spiritual and the sacred. Thus, Native American religion and spirituality is entirely cultural. One does not "convert" to this religion any more than one "converts" to being Native American. Second, due to a history of long-term contact with missions and Christian influences, many Native Americans are Christian while also holding onto traditional tribal beliefs.

History

One of the first treaties between the United States and American Indians was made in 1778 between the United States on one side and Captain White Eyes, Captain John Kill Buck, and Captain Pipe on the other. It was a treaty established for the purposes of peaceful passage through Native Territory and to assure the indigenous people that there was no intent to "take possession of their country." Article I states that "All offences or acts of hostilities by one, or either of the contracting parties against the other, be mutually forgiven, and buried in the depth of oblivion, never more to be had in remembrance" (*Treaty with the Delawares: 1778*, Yale Law School n.d.). It was about respect and possession. What was not understood at the time by those marking "x" as their signatures, or by those who could write, was that this Article about respect and possession was only the beginning of devastation for the American Indians. Treaty-making ended by 1871, and from 1887 to 1934 the United States government promoted assimilation by prohibiting American Indian ceremonies and promoting English boarding school education.

In 1822, Jedediah Morse published a report for the purposes of "awakening the attention ... to the state of this neglected and oppressed people" by counting American Indians and identifying where they lived (Morse 1822: 9). The real awakening should have come with the disease and death taking place by the mid-1800s. Smallpox killed thousands of indigenous people, in some cases wiping out entire groups. According to Henry Rowe Schoolcraft, "Language, however forcible, fails to give an idea of the reality" (Schoolcraft 1857). By the end of the nineteenth century, there were approximately 250,000 American Indians (estimates of the population at the time of European encroachment range between 1.2 and 12 million).

In 1921, through the Bureau of Indian Affairs, the federal government encouraged the use of force to halt religious practices that would hinder assimilation, but by 1928, the assimilation project was declared a failure, and religious and cultural practices were soon considered legal. In the 1970s, the US government returned some sacred lands to the American Indians (a sacred lake to the Taos Pueblo Indians and a portion of Mount Adams to the Yakama Indians), but struggles for religious freedoms continued through the 1980s and 1990s over issues such as control of sacred lands, exercise of religious and cultural practices prohibited by other laws (substances used in ceremonies, etc.), the protection of knowledge (sacred and general) from exploitation, and the control of human remains and sacred objects held in museums.

When the Natives were relegated to vast tracts of land, the wound was not just to the American Indians themselves. In their minds, the earth was wounded, which meant that they as caretakers of the earth were also wounded at a very deep, soul level. In relegating the American Indians to reservations, the US government assumed certain responsibilities, one of which was the provision of health services, but there was little understanding of the depth and spiritual nature of the wound (Rhoades 2000). By 1849, the Office of Indian Affairs dealt mostly with health on the reservations and provided minimal health services. By the beginning of the twentieth century, it seemed that the indigenous population would continue to dwindle; however, within the second half of the twentieth century there was a fivefold increase in the population due to rising birth rates, declining mortality, increasing numbers of people identifying as American Indian and Alaska Native, who also identify themselves in other groups (Rhoades 2000). Questions emerged around what qualifies a person to be Native American. For my father, he was American Indian because both his mother and father "were half American Indian." His identity was defined by what he "felt," understood, and where he had a sense of belonging. But more technical questions emerged around blood quantum rules (for example, original Alaska Native shareholders had to be one-quarter or more) and tribal enrollment restrictions and cutoff dates, all of which affect indigenous belonging and grouping (National Public Radio 2022; Alaskan Natives n.d.).

In 1955, the Indian Health Service (IHS) was established and now serves members of American Indian tribes throughout the country. It also funds contracts, such as one in Southern California called the Riverside-San Bernardino County Indian Health, Inc. (rsbcihi.org), which is a tribally managed healthcare organization comprised of a consortium of ten tribes. There is also an *Alaska Native Tribal Health Consortium* that provides health services to Alaska Native people (www.anthc.org/). Among the goals of both are to provide culturally appropriate healthcare services by respecting and abiding by customs and traditions and to promote wellness by striving to provide state-of-the-art healthcare. Through this complex organization of community-oriented primary care, American

Indians receive basic healthcare. One of the challenges is that, while Native Americans are eligible for this care, many move away from the reservations into metropolitan areas and reside outside the scope of IHS and tribal care systems (Snipp 2000: 56). Currently, the comprehensive health service delivery system of the IHS agency serves 2.56 million patients (Indian Health Service 2020b).

Another factor complicates healthcare delivery. The American Indian elder is a position of leadership based on wisdom, community service, and experience, rather than chronological age. The community group may refer to someone as young as 40 or in their early 50s as an "elder." They are the ones most closely connected to a painful historical past on one hand, and the heroic oral histories on the other. They are the keepers of the sacred songs that often are not allowed to be taped and studied by outsiders. The younger generations sometimes go to them for health remedies, either before seeking medical care or after Western modern medicine has failed. In contrast, from the perspective of the Indian Health Service, an American Indian elder is someone 55 years of age or older. For healthcare givers within the IHS, American Indian elders are simply the aging group within the American Indian population – older versions of the young, rather than keepers of a rich tradition (Deloria 1997).

The term "tribal sovereignty" suggests that Native tribes/nations have the authority to govern themselves, which means that, in general, the states have no legal jurisdiction in Native country, or reservation territory. Indigenous tribes can make laws affecting conduct, enforce laws through tribal police, exclude non-members from the reservation, and regulate environmental protection. This idea of sovereignty creates complexities in the way American Indians relate to the federal government on issues connected to healthcare (Kim 2008).

Beliefs and practices

General

American Indians have a different way of thinking when they are within traditional cultural contexts and natural environments, notes Donald Fixico, a leading American Indian historian. He argues that Native thinking is "visual and circular in philosophy," suggesting that it is a combination of two realities – the physical and the metaphysical (Fixico 2003: xii). Decision making is a response to listening and observing the natural environment and then balancing all factors in the process of coming to a consensus. "The right decision is the best decision for all concerned" (Fixico 2003: xii). Of particular interest is the concept of "listening" and "seeing." "Listening" has less to do with sounds than with gaining information for understanding the connections and their meanings. "Seeing" is visualizing all the possible connections and their relationships with each other. It is viewing from a holistic perspective. For example, with my father's skin cancer, my primary concern was his nose, and whether or not the skin changes were actually cancer. For my father, it had more to do with his life, his desire to know the actual medical diagnosis (or not to know it), his relation to nature and natural healing, how the current moment might play out in the future, and the process of making a decision. For him it was about the whole, and all the connections that go with that. Thus, "seeing" and "listening" make up Native thinking.

With the circular way of thinking found in the indigenous mind, there are not two focal points; there is only one, and all illustrations reflect on that one point with the purpose of increasing understanding and the possibility for harmony. The non-indigenous mind is more linear, proceeding from point A to point B and valuing empirical evidence more highly than the story. In linear thinking, the purpose is to pursue goals, work hard, look to the future, and not be distracted by those around you.

Circular thinking is all about the capacity to look in all directions and appreciate everything that one sees. At the center of this circle is peace – a sacred space of rest, balance, and wholeness that defies the chaos going on around it. Sickness is being out of balance, of failing to see the connections, of having no peace at the center. In this way, religion and medicine connect. Both address issues of balance, harmony, and wholeness. While most American Indians have been educated in mainstream schools, many still "see" from this indigenous non-linear perspective, and this has implications for healthcare (Fixico 2003: xii).

While this form of thinking does characterize the American Indian "mindset" in general, each tribe is different, each is unique. In comparison to the typical North American mindset, however, American Indians can be said to consider life to be sacred. Some feel themselves to be "holy people" and to be "called to live a holy life." Rituals and ceremonies are essential, as are those who conduct them. These shamans or "medicine men (or women)" also help the community to maintain traditional healing practices. Oral traditions remain strong, thus there is no written scripture in their religions. Relationship with the land is very important to most American Indians, which is deeply related to the experience of religion. In the end, at death, Natives often believe they "go to God." Some Native American beliefs are more universal, such as reverence and respect for life and the belief that all things are sacred – even rocks, plants, and dust. Another belief shared by most tribes is that death is a part of life and is not from God (or any other deity) but happens to all people once they have fulfilled the purpose for life. Another common belief is that to be healthy is to be in balance – mind, body, and spirit. Other beliefs are unique to the particular tribe of American Indians. Some tribes have restrictions on what they can look at. Some believe in ghosts, while others do not. Many tribes practice a similar ceremony, such as the sun dance, while practicing it differently.

What the tribes share is the belief in the sacredness of all things and people. While not all tribes describe themselves as a "holy people," they share the belief that their lives are infused with the spiritual – that life is about balance and the connection of all things. A common Lakota salutation and saying at the end of a prayer illustrates this respect and connectedness of all things – *Mitakuye Oyasin*, meaning "to all my relations," which includes family, extended family, and nature as well. The relevance of family and community to indigenous people has been grossly underestimated, with various healthcare disciplines trying to better understand the value of family and community as cornerstones in Native American culture (Swanson et al. 2021). People, mountains, and bodies of water are all sacred beings and also make up the family, about which the American Indian cares deeply.

There are a variety of ceremonies and rituals. Some tribes allow children to be present during healing rituals (Lakota), believing that friends and family help restore the ill to balance, and some do not allow the presence of children (Apache). The purpose of the medicine men and women is to counteract the supernatural forces as much as possible. They refer to those who practice indigenous healing that focuses on physical healing, spiritual healing, or both (Sutton & Nose 2005). These traditional healers understand the connections between nature and health and often use ceremonies to determine the cause and treatment of disease. These ceremonies can take up to several days. Natural or traditional remedies include the use of herb medicines, special rituals, and sweat lodges (heated dome-shaped structures in which Native people have spiritual experiences). The use of traditional remedies illustrates the sense of connectedness with the natural world and the belief that one should live in harmony with it.

Some songs and prayers that accompany the ceremonies are secret, and those who know the songs must be present for the ceremonies to take place. This highlights the importance of the oral tradition of the Native American. The oral tradition begins with the telling of various creation stories, depending on the tribal tradition. Stories vary from an androgynous creator figure (for Zunis) to a stronger twin brother (for many Native American cultures), or to a suffering hero figure (for Navajos). Among most tribes, however, there is the sense of a single creative force, which manifests itself in everything human and non-human. That creative force grants spirit-power to animals and other non-human entities. The stories also explore the notion of four directions, which must be in balance for health to be possible.

Native American myths contain all types of genres, including trickster myths such as Coyote and Iktome, who bring forth humans, while at the same time causing problems for them. This commitment to the oral tradition helped to preserve knowledge. It also preserved a flexibility that allowed the Native American to survive a variety of threats by integrating foreign aspects without losing itself.

American Indians are often passionate about protecting "Mother Earth" because she is "life itself." This religious or spiritual regard for the land typifies the way in which the American Indian connects with space rather than the more typical time-orientation of most Americans. It also suggests that while many Native Americans may be Christian, they often still connect to native spirituality. American Indians in general, regardless of the tribe or perspectives on Christianity, believe in the sacredness of the land – both general and particular. All land is sacred in that they are to live in harmony with it and not destroy it. In addition, particular lands are sacred in that American Indians have a particular commitment to take care of *that* land – to fish and hunt with ethical commitments to the moral standing of all that lives within it. Traditionally, the Native American communicated with the Creator through interacting with the natural elements of animals, plants, and nature in general. Many were given symbolic animals (names, symbols) to reflect their own human characteristics, or with the hopes that these animal spirits would infuse their animal characteristics into the individual. In this way, fishing, hunting, religion, and the land are all interconnected in ways that are inseparable.

In conclusion, to understand Native American beliefs and practices, we must "listen" and "see" through non-linear thinking rather than linear, empirical thinking. To accomplish this, narrative and storytelling are the preferred methods for the discussion, as well as exploring a variety of metaphors. In the introduction to his book, *Healing the Soul Wound*, Eduardo Duran, himself an American Indian and a psychologist working in Indian territory, explains that he faced the decision of whether to "embroider the fabric of the clinical work with academic language and theoretical constructs or simply say what needs to be said" (Duran 2006: 1). In the end, he decided simply to present the story. If we listen well, it may be necessary to modify or change some Western practices in order to better serve the American Indian population (Duran 2006).

Health and disease

Keith is a 32-year-old American Indian man who lives in an urban area and works as a salesman in a small hobby shop during the day and as a cabinetmaker in the evening. He has little contact with his tribal culture, occasionally participating in cultural events on a reservation located an hour's drive from where he lives. During a visit to his local physician for a diabetes check-up, he confesses that he is struggling with alcohol and wonders if he is depressed. He tells the story of picking up his gun and holding it to his chest, imagining that all the pain in his life is over. Laughingly he states, "Maybe I should get some bee stingers from the Elder. Maybe that would help."

In order to understand and address Keith's situation, some background will help. American Indians and Alaska Natives living in the United States have a lower health status than the average American. They have lower life expectancy by 9.9 years (67.1 years compared to 77.0 for the average American) and higher infant mortality rates (7.59 out of 1,000 deaths compared to 5.39 out of 1,000 deaths) (Arias & Xu 2022).

There are higher rates of many sexually transmitted diseases such as gonorrhea, chlamydia, and syphilis (Centers for Disease Control and Prevention 2020). The leading cause of death in those aged 10–44 is unintentional injury, the second leading cause of death (ages 10–44) is suicide, the third is liver disease or cancer (depending on age), and the fourth is homicide. In those aged 45–85, the first and second leading causes of death are heart disease and cancer (Centers for Disease Control and Prevention 2017). In relation to mental health services, there is a lack of funding and a high turnover of mental health professionals, and the mental health services are often not culturally appropriate. For these reasons, mental health services are often underutilized (Gone 2004: 10–18).

This background helps us understand Keith better. Given the tendency not to utilize mental health services, he confesses his psychological issues to his physician. Suicide is the second leading cause of death in his age category, with unintentional injury being the first, so his thoughts of suicide should not surprise us. He has little connection to his tribal culture, so in some ways he is disconnected from his past, and perhaps experiences disconnection in general, enhancing the feeling of depression.

Keith brings more than personal depression. He brings with him generations of stories related to suffering. The relation between historical events and current constructions of health/illness is both relevant and complex in the healing encounter. The concept of intergenere. This concept suggests that the trauma that is not dealt with in a previous generation is passed down to the next generation to deal with and may become more

Table 4.1 American Indian and Alaska Native mortality rates for specific diseases compared with all races in the U.S.

Disease	AI/AN Rate 2009–2011	Ratio: AI/AN to U.S. All Races
Alcoholism	50	6.6
Liver Disease	43	4.6
Diabetes	66	3.2
Accidents	94	2.5
Homicide	11	2.1
Suicide	20	1.7

Source: Indian Health Service (2020a)

severe as it passes down (Nebelkopf & Phillips 2004). This trauma may be internalized and expressed as domestic and/or institutional violence. The American Indian considers historical trauma, or intergenerational trauma, as a wound to the soul or spirit, referred to by some as a "soul wound," giving it "spiritual dimensions" (Duran 2006). In this sense, Keith brings more than individual depression. He brings a historical context that is deeply connected to the soul or spirit, and this affects the clinical encounter.

Finally, while Keith has little connection to his tribal culture, it continues to inform him, and thus he explores the concept of traditional healing. Traditional healing practices often treat the person holistically, treating the physical body as well as the soul. His reference to a traditional healing practice suggests the ways in which Western and traditional healing practices may overlap. If Keith were to subscribe entirely to traditional practices, he might enter a formal ceremony for healing, with burning plants, throwing cornmeal, or using bee stingers to treat disease. What is less understood by the current physician is that while Keith questions the use of bee stingers as treatment, his deeper desire is that the current physician treats him from a holistic perspective – that his soul and his body are connected and unless his spirit is in harmony with the rest, little else matters.

Helping Keith manage his illness demands attention to many factors. The first is to the non-linear and narrative emphasis in the American Indian mindset. Emerging from his current sense of depression will require a new story. But before a new narrative can begin, the old one must be understood, and this involves understanding the "soul wound." In trying to understand the historical context, the practitioner can ask the following question: "Where did you learn how to do this?" This can be followed up with, "And where did *they* learn how to do this?"

The practitioner must also be aware of his or her own historical context and the complexities this might bring. In speaking of the American Indians, one female Caucasian physician stated, "Just by virtue of being Caucasian, I am sometimes initially viewed as the enemy." It is helpful when practitioners are in touch with and aware of their own woundedness. This also suggests that healing is not dependent on someone in a higher position or on the medical model itself, but that healing has something to do with understanding the dichotomy within oneself – a sort of harmonizing of opposites. Again, this idea undercuts the view that illness is simply a pathologized self and comes closer to a traditional Indian view that healing has to do with harmonizing various, even opposing, elements.

One's own historical context also affects transference which, in the world of the American Indian, can be interpreted literally as energy transferring from one person to another – both negative and positive, depending on the practitioner's attitudes toward the Native, and on whether one has worked out one's own personal history. If the practitioner is an American Indian, he or she must avoid the belief that by belonging to the same group, there is automatic understanding (Duran 2006).

Viewing the treatment of illness as a ceremony that has specific physical or metaphorical boundaries may also help move Keith toward a new, healthier story. For example, the office may be the "container" in which the healing ceremony takes place. Instead of smoke and cornmeal, there may be other objects with which an American Indian can identify – pictures, artwork, objects related to healing. Making a diagnosis is a part of this ceremony – the naming of illness. Identifying a diagnosis for the American Indian can be viewed as a type of naming ceremony, where spiritual identities accompany the name. For the American Indian, illness has its own consciousness and works out a

purpose within the body to restore it to wholeness. It is not so much the goal to overcome illness as it is to have a relationship with it, to understand its purpose, and to har-
monize with it. A diagnosis may not be perceived by the American Indian as something
to "treat" or "conquer" as much as it is to be understood and harmonized. The root
metaphor of illness for the indigenous person is closer to relationship than pathology
(Duran 2006).

A useful model for such clinical interactions has been developed by Lakota tribal
leader Gene Thin Elk. He has designed an indigenous, culturally specific model called
The Red Road to Recovery, which has helped thousands of people toward the creation of
a healthier personal story. This model works from a holistic perspective and incorporates
many traditional practices that make healing relevant and sensitive to the needs of the
American Indian population. This reconnecting of American Indians to their cultural
background takes seriously an important and essential past. Rather than teaching the
American Indian how to be more Westernized, the model suggests that the healthcare
practitioner must learn to speak Red (Nebelkopf & Phillips 2004). Learning to speak
Red might mean becoming familiar with local resources that are sensitive to the needs
of the American Indian. It might also mean incorporating such resources into one's own
practice.

It is important to note the degree to which American Indians identify with their traditional culture. Knowing whether they live on a reservation and the degree of belief in and
contact with traditional practices is important. Keith is not unusual. Diabetes and depression are major health problems among American Indians. What surprises the physician
is that when Keith attempts to describe the cause of his diabetes, in a quiet gentle voice
he begins to reflect on the history of the American Indian, rather than on his personal
history. According to him, his people have left the old ways of healing and adopted the
foods of the White world, and this is why he has diabetes. He explains his attempts
to eat more traditional foods. What has previously appeared to the physician as non-
compliance is actually a man trying to come to terms with his own history. He attempts
to be connected to the past, and to restore it.

The American Indian's (re-)claiming of traditional foods and dietary taboos can take
different forms, depending on the tribe and tradition. Traditionally, the issue has not been
about what foods one is allowed to eat, but rather a focus on foods that create *wicozani*
(Sioux word) or balance. Processed meats, sugared drinks, the lack of fresh produce, and
easy access to drugs and alcohol have contributed to many and various health problems
among American Indians, such as diabetes, obesity, and substance abuse. Following the
medicine wheel, which has four sections representing the four natural elements, they seek
balance among four food types – water, meat, gathered plants, and cultivated plants,
which should be consumed in equal portions. When one returns to a more traditional
way of eating in such a manner, balance and healing can occur.

The juxtaposition between the traditional and the modern can also be seen in the area
of procreation and sexual morality. As with other attitudes, Native American attitudes
about contraception have a history. Native American women have had hundreds of years
of experience using natural, traditional contraceptive methods, such as not having sex
during the most fertile times, using crushed roots of red cedar and juniper plants in
teas, or making concoctions from other plants to prevent births, some of which are used
in commercial products for oral contraceptives (Mexican wild yam). American Indians
have also used plant substances to induce abortions and cause sterility. As for the use of

commercial contraceptives, Native American women's attitudes vary. Many do not use them, influenced by their husbands, extended family, or historical concerns. In general, tribal traditions tend to work against the use of commercial contraceptives, although this is changing and is partially dependent on a woman's age and number of children.

On the issue of abortion, Native American traditional health practices include the use of plants (black cohosh, black snakeroot, and squaw root) to stimulate the uterus, cause menstruation, or induce abortion. Native American cultures also believe that family planning is a part of respecting Mother Earth, with many Native American women feeling that decisions for abortion lay within their sphere, instead of the sphere of men or governmental agencies or laws. At the same time, because of the sacred value that they place upon the life cycle that begins and continues through conception and pregnancy and the preference that they have for natural and traditional means, American Indians have generally been averse to the invasive abortion procedures carried out in Western clinical settings, leading some tribes to ban modern abortion procedures altogether from clinics on Indian reservations.

Not surprisingly, those in the modern Western world are not as familiar with the value of connections with the past. American Indian *connection* suffers from dislocation from native lands, weakened parental influence due to mission and boarding schools, and weakened cultural ties. The healthcare professional should explore ways to re-establish these protective factors. For example, Lakota children are *wakanheja* or sacred, and taking care of these children is a sacred responsibility for both parents and the community (Nebelkopf & Phillips 2004). The idea of family may not only refer to the nuclear family, but may often extend to clans and lineages, revealing systems of loyalties that are critical. In this way, the community joins together to take care of its own. Putting the American Indian back in contact with his or her own cultural values of connection is more important than trying to instill "modern" values.

Death and dying

According to one American Indian myth, death exists because Coyote prevented the chief medicine man from catching death (portrayed as a whirlwind), so death continues to roam the earth. While this would seem to make death fearful, few American Indians fear death because of their belief that all things are interdependent. American Indians view death as a journey that proceeds beyond death, with ancestral spirits returning to interact with the living. It is a natural part of life.

While most tribes believe in a spiritual journey to the afterlife, some have a fear of ghosts (Navajo and Apache), while others do not (Hopi). The Apache believe that the spirit hangs around after death and a person can get "ghost sickness" by touching a dead body. The Alaska Native has no conception of a supreme spirit, although ancestral spirits may come to the family. Others suggest that disease-causing agents can take the form of snakes or owls and enter our dreams, creating havoc or causing illness. Most tribes believe that illness might be incurred from handling a deceased body. Some remain present while a loved one is dying; others do not. Some tribes tie prayer feathers to the hair and each foot of the deceased to aid them in their journey to the afterlife.

While the suicide rates are high for American Indians, the traditional belief does not support it, suggesting that those who commit suicide wander aimlessly on the earth (Cox 2003). In one study of American Indians living on reservations, a strong protective factor against suicide was tribal spiritual orientation, or forms of spirituality derived from traditions that predate European contact (referred to as "cultural spirituality") (Garroutte et al. 2003: 1571–1579). Traditional healing practices look at a person holistically, thus they address the soul as well as the physical body. When American Indians seek traditional health practices it may be this holistic perspective that they desire, and this perspective is often missing in Western medicine. Where the American Indian understands the connection between a troubled soul and a diseased body, Western medicine often denies, or at least fails to address, this connection.

Funeral concerns vary from tribe to tribe. Some tribes (Navajo) shun the body and effects of the deceased, believing that the ghost stays behind. They believe that the body should be buried quickly, while a wake may last for several days (called "sings"). Other tribes (Lakota) believe that the body can be held for a period of time before burial. Since families are matriarchal, generally it is the wife, mother, or grandmother of the deceased who makes the arrangements for burial. The family may want to transport the body to the home of the deceased and paint the face according to the tribe. Burial and cremation are both allowed, depending on the tribe. Sometimes family and friends help dig the grave, referred to as "The Dig."

At the funeral ceremony, often an elder presides and a funeral director is not involved at all. The ceremony may include drumming and singing, and a feast in honor of the deceased, and may continue through the night(s). Many Native Americans place personal items belonging to the deceased, such as clothes and blankets, in the grave. There is the belief that everything made has the spirit of the maker in it, thus they often cut or break the item to release that spirit. For this reason, often broken pottery surrounds the gravesite. Sometimes, even the end of the casket is left unsealed in order to allow the spirit to be released.

After the funeral is grief and, according to Native American culture, there are many lessons about grief, its duration, and what can grow out of grief. In the Shoshone legend of the Caterpillar People, a dying caterpillar man leaves behind a grieving caterpillar woman. She grieves for a year until Great Mystery tells her that it is time to stop, at which point she turns into a butterfly and brings the world beauty, grace, and color.

The most important thing is that those who help Native American families plan funerals need to respect Native traditions and work in cooperation with their spiritual leaders. Native Americans approach death with awe, reverence, and love for the departed, as well as a fear that knowledge about their beliefs may be used to their disadvantage, thus there may be some reticence on the subject. It would be helpful for the healthcare practitioner to understand this.

Conclusion

For the healthcare practitioner to treat patients such as Keith, there must be some understanding of his culture and religion, as well as his historical context. This takes time, which is why trust is not quickly or easily built. Keith's healthcare practitioner can treat him without fully understanding him, but the treatment will never approach what is necessary for Keith to find true healing. Keith's pain is larger than his current context. The naming of his "disease" will not be captured by the terms "diabetic" or "suicidal" or "depression." His disconnection will not be remedied by a prescription for medication. As is true in the case of my father, "next time" he may do something different. With Keith, there may not even be another "next time." To speak in the language of the

Table 4.2 Dos and don'ts

Dos	Don'ts
1. Recognize that illness and health are spiritually oriented and not just physiological pathology.	1. Do not treat the patient like a number; a creature present in your clinic that needs something you can give.
2. As the caregiver, try to allow yourself a deep and present emersion into your own sense of what it means to be a whole, unitive person who is ill. Be a "wounded healer."	2. Do not allow yourself to slide into being a cold, detached technician.
3. Create and fully incorporate as many ways as possible of connecting with the patient. Include the use of the creative arts, metaphors, storytelling, dreams, and play.	3. Do not maintain those elements of your practice that put distance between you and your patient.
4. Effective connection must include understanding the story the patient has to tell, including the historical story. Stick with it, listen to it, and hear it.	4. Do not allow yourself to be distracted. When you are with your patient, be fully present.
5. In this connection, a kind of ceremonial connection, work with the patient to identify and name the illness.	5. Do not foist upon the patient a technical and complicated diagnosis or find and identify the illness without collaboration with the patient.
6. Begin then to create a new story that incorporates as much as possible the traditional, cultural ways to return the patient to health.	6. Do not rush out of the appointment. Providing culturally sensitive care sometimes takes more time than you expect.
	7. Do not demand to practice modern Western medicine without being influenced or taught by traditional healing ways.
	8. Do not avoid being touched by the individual and the historical story.

American Indian is not just to make the notation of "American Indian" in the patient's chart; it is to understand that the notation represents an entire history, a rich tradition, a deep connection with the land, a tradition of storytelling, and the infusion of sacredness in everything from children to the natural elements. To speak in the language of the American Indian is to realize the breadth and depth of woundedness as well as healing, the value of circular thinking, and the importance of an inner core of peace and harmony. It is to ask, "Can you tell me more about . . .," not just for the purposes of understanding, but for the purposes of learning. Listening is an act of humility and by placing oneself in the position of not knowing one can be taught.

Case study #1

A nurse at the regional trauma hospital was reviewing pre-surgery consent forms with her patient, a male of Cherokee heritage, in his late 50s. He had suffered from poorly controlled diabetes for 20 years, resulting in peripheral artery disease and neuropathy. After falling, a wound on his lower leg never healed properly and slowly became gangrenous. The patient now needed a below-the-knee amputation.

After his nurse explained the procedure and recovery process, the patient was reticent to sign the consent for surgery. He wanted to take his amputated leg home with him. The nurse was new and surprised by his request. It seemed unsanitary to her. When she spoke to her charge nurse, she learned that, as the regional hospital that served a Cherokee reservation, there was a hospital policy that allowed for patients to retrieve their amputated limbs. She explained that the policy was developed out of respect for religions that believe a person must be buried with all of their body parts.

The charge nurse came to speak with the patient and explained that there would be an additional form from Risk Management that would need to be completed and sent to the Pathology department where the limb would be processed according to lab and legal statutes. The patient's removed leg would be ready for him two weeks after the surgery. The patient visibly relaxed when he heard this news and signed both the consent forms, now ready for the procedure.

Questions for reflection

1. What do you imagine will be done with the amputated limb once the patient takes it home?
2. Why might this particular hospital have such a policy? Why might a hospital have reservations about this?
3. What other religions besides Native Americans would feel it important to be buried with all their limbs?
4. What implications might this type of belief system have for patients that are potential organ donors?

*Submitted by Niesha Steinke

Case study #2

A 28-year-old female member of the Navajo Nation with end stage liver failure arrives at the ER in a critical access hospital in the Southwest. With an extremely poor prognosis, there was little more to do for her than to keep her comfortable as she died. Her family lived ten hours away but drove to be with her in her last moments. The patient died on the night her family arrived. Some of her family wanted to perform traditional religious customs including chanting, singing, smudging, and the burning of sage. Since hospital fire codes prohibit burning, the smudging and sage burning in the patient's room were not permitted. The singing and chanting were easily accommodated by the nursing staff. The family also helped the nurses with the final cleansing of her body. Coordinating with the day shift staffing and management, they arranged to take her body outdoors to a special little garden on the grounds of the hospital so that the final rituals of smudging and burning of sage could take place.

The nurses and supervisors believe they made every effort to accommodate the wishes of the family within the scope of hospital regulations. One nurse recognized that "being able to acknowledge and allow the customs of patients within the acute care setting is challenging at times and important for all parties involved." Sometimes the issues we face in clinical healthcare push us outside our comfort zone. The nurse went on to say: "By thinking outside the box for creative solutions we were able to honor the requests of the family members at least to some extent."

Questions for reflection

1. Evaluate the actions of the nursing staff and hospital administration in their "thinking outside the box," including accommodating the noise in the patient's room from

the singing and dancing. How might the burning of sage in the patient's room have endangered the safety of others?
2. Kits for smudging are widely available for purchase from non-Native American sources. What are the pros and cons of this cultural appropriation for commercial purposes?
3. Religions often call for specific end of life rituals on behalf of dying and deceased patients. How can healthcare administrators best prepare their staff for these diverse needs?

*Submitted by Kimberly Martin

Glossary

American Indian/Native American Indigenous people as well as those who study, research, and write on American Indians use the terms interchangeably.
Mitakuye Oyasin A common Lakota salutation and saying at the end of a prayer illustrates the respect for and connectedness of all things. Means literally, "to all my relations."
Story/storytelling In the mind of the American Indian, the purpose of the story is to define, create, and understand reality. The story, storytelling, and folklore are primary elements in maintaining tradition, preserving knowledge, and protecting the truth of the past for the American Indian.
Sweat lodge or "inipi" Generally it takes place in a hut or mostly enclosed area and water is poured over hot rocks so that steam rises, creating a sauna-like effect. It often occurs before and after all other ceremonies or is used as a stand-alone ceremony to cleanse or purify.
Traditional healing Traditional healing includes the traditions around health and illness not based on Western science but on tribal beliefs about how to live. Each tribe has its own methods and materials put to use in these traditional healing techniques.

Note

1 Roy Kim, one of the original authors of this chapter, was unable to be involved in the update for this third edition.

Bibliography

Abram, D. (2010) *Becoming Animal: An Earthly Cosmology*. New York: Pantheon.
Acutrans (2020) *Indigenous Languages of the United States*. www.acutrans.com/indigenous-languages-of-the-united-states
Alaskan Natives (n.d.) www.alaskan-natives.com/333/major-indian-tribes-alaska *Alaska Natives' Complicated Identities*. Part I: https://alaskapublic.org/2021/07/15/alaska-natives-complica ted-identities/ Part II: https://alaskapublic.org/2021/07/28/the-next-generation-of-alaska-native-shareholders/
Arias, E. and Xu, J. (2022) "United States Life Tables, 2020," *National Vital Statistics Reports*, 71(1).
Centeno, J. (2021) "10 Biggest Native American Tribes Today," *Native American Nations*. www.powwows.com/10-biggest-native-american-tribes-today
Centers for Disease Control and Prevention (2017) Leading Causes of Death-Males-Non-Hispanic American Indian or Alaska Native-United States, 2017. www.cdc.gov/healthequity/lcod/men/2017/nonhispanic-native/index.htm

Centers for Disease Control and Prevention (2020) *Health Disparities in HIV, Viral Hepatitis, SDSs, and TB: American Indians and Alaska Natives.* www.cdc.gov/nchhstp/healthdisparities/americanindians.html

Cohen, F. (1982) *Handbook of Federal Indian Law.* Charlottesville, VA: Michie Co.

Cox, G. (2003) "The Native American way of death," in Bryant, C. (ed.) *Handbook of Death and Dying: Volume Two: The Response to Death.* Thousand Oaks, CA: Sage Publications.

Deloria Jr., V. (1997) *Red Earth, White Lies: Native Americans and the Myth of Scientific Fact.* Golden, CO: Fulcrum Publishing.

Duran, E. (2006) *Healing the Soul Wound: Counseling with American Indians and Other Native Peoples.* New York: Teachers College Press.

Fixico, D. (2003) *The American Indian Mind in a Linear World.* New York: Routledge.

Garroutte, E., Goldberg, J., Herrell, R., and Manson, S. (2003) "Spirituality and attempted suicide among American Indians," *Social Science & Medicine,* 56(7): 1571–1579.

Gone, J. (2004) "Mental health services for Native Americans in the 21st century United States," *Professional Psychology: Research and Practice,* 35: 10–18.

Gustafson, F. (1997) *Dancing Between Two Worlds: Jung and the Native American Soul.* New York: Paulist Press.

Indian Health Service (2020a) *Disparities.* www.ihs.gov/newsroom/factsheets/disparities/

Indian Health Service (2020b) *IHS Profile.* www.ihs.gov/newsroom/factsheets/ihsprofile/

Kim, R. (2008) Personal visit at the Morongo Indian Reservation, San Bernardino County, California, November 21, 2008.

Lakota Sioux Chief Yellow Lark (Trans.) (1887) *Native American Prayers: Great Spirit Prayer.* www.xavier.edu/jesuitresource/online-resources/prayer-index/native-american

Marya, R. and Patel, RAJ., (2021) *Inflamed: Deep Medicine and the Anatomy of Injustice.* New York: Farrar, Straus, and Giroux.

Morse, J. (1822) *A Report to the Secretary of War of the United States on Indian Affairs 1822.* Washington, DC: Davis & Force.

National Congress of American Indians (2020) *Tribal Nations & the United States: An Introduction.* https://ncai.org/about-tribes

National Public Radio (2022) *The Nooksack Tribe in Washington is Attempting to Evict People from Their Tribal Homes,* Weekend Edition, December 11, 2022. www.npr.org/2022/12/11/1142119438/the-nooksack-tribe-in-washington-is-attempting-to-evict-people-from-tribal-homes

Nebelkopf, E. and Phillips, M. (eds.) (2004) *Healing and Mental Health for Native Americans: Speaking in Red.* New York: Altamira Press.

Public Religion Research Institute (2021) The 2020 Census of American Religion. www.prri.org/research/2020-census-of-american-religion/

Rhoades, E. (ed.) (2000) *American Indian Health: Innovations in Healthcare, Promotion, and Policy.* London: Johns Hopkins University Press.

Riverside San Bernardino County Indian Health (RSBCIHI) (n.d.) www.rsbcihi.org

Schoolcraft, HR. (1857) *History of the Indian Tribes of the United States: Their Present Condition and Prospects, and a Sketch of their Ancient Status.* Philadelphia, PA: J. B. Lippincott.

Snipp, CM. (2000) "Selected demographic characteristics of Indians," in Rhoades, E. (ed.) *American Indian Health: Innovations in Healthcare, Promotion, and Policy* (pp. 41–60). London: Johns Hopkins University Press.

Spector, R. (2000) *Cultural Diversity in Health and Illness.* Upper Saddle River, NJ: Prentice Hall Health.

Sutton, C. and Nose, M. (2005) "American Indian Families," in McGoldrick, M., Giordano, J., and Garcia-Preto, N. (eds) *Ethnicity & Family Therapy* (pp. 43–54). New York: The Guilford Press.

Swanson, S., Nygard, R., and Saus, M. (2021). "Native American Social Work – Including Family and Community," *Journal of Social Work*, 22(3): 615–636. https://doi.org/10.1177/146801 73211009177

US Census Bureau (2021) *Facts for Features: American Indian and Alaska Native Heritage Month: November 2021*. www.census.gov/newsroom/facts-for-features/2021/aian-month.html

Yale Law School, Lillian Goldman Law Library (n.d.) Treaty with the Delawares: 1778. http://ava lon.law.yale.edu/18th_century/del1778.asp

5 Hinduism

Manoj Shah[1] and Siroj Sorajjakool

Fear not what is not real, never was, and never will be. What is real, always was and cannot be destroyed.

(*Bhagavad Gita* 2007: 2:16)

Introduction

Hinduism, the third largest religion in the world, represents a collection of beliefs, practices, and ethos that arose in India around 1500 BCE. It is rooted in the *Vedas* and the history of the people of India and connected by *sanatana dharma*, "eternal duty," which suggests a common orientation toward liberation from the cycle of birth and rebirth (Young 2005: 58–59).

The term Hinduism is in itself complex and requires careful analysis so as to represent it more accurately. The religion that we now call Hinduism has "no historical founder, no single scriptural text recognized by all, no single authoritative voice or organization or institution, no common creed" (Schmidt et al. 1999: 208). While the history of Hinduism may be traced back to 1500 BCE, the designation "Hindu" was used much later and referred to the people of the Indus Valley. This new designation came as an attempt to create a religious distinction when Islam came to India.

Another complication with the term Hinduism is the diversity of beliefs and practices found within the religion. There are many gods with various ritual beliefs and practices. Despite these many variations of beliefs and practices, the common thread that holds things together appears to be the social traditions of those who follow Hinduism. Prakash Desai, professor of clinical psychiatry at the University of Illinois, explains:

Perhaps here lies the secret of the survival of the Hindu tradition. Accumulating various interpretations of reality, Hindus arrive at a vision of the good life determined by adaptation and accommodation to prevailing conditions. As the subcultures of multiple ethnic groups were being assimilated into a social order, regulation of behavior appears to have been more important than regulation of beliefs. The private lives of the populace were left alone, and in early India few attempts were made at consolidating a social philosophy that would then govern both public and private behavior. The result is a profound conviction that "truth" or self-realization is discovered through many paths, and a simultaneous rejection of absolutes in consideration of personal morality.

(Desai 1989: 11)

DOI: 10.4324/9781003288862-5

Hence the diversity of beliefs and practices are closely connected to the social traditions of the people of the Indus Valley creating unity within these variations, which is now called Hinduism.

Demographics

There are approximately 1.2 billion Hindus in the world, comprising roughly 15 percent of the world population. The three nations with the highest percentage of Hindu population are India, Nepal, and Mauritius with significant numbers in the following countries: Bangladesh, Indonesia (especially Bali), Sri Lanka, Pakistan, Indonesia, and other Southeast Asian countries such as Malaysia, Singapore, and Thailand. There are one billion Hindus in India or approximately 78.9 percent of the total population. The United States has the seventh largest Hindu population at 2.51 million comprising 0.7 percent of the US population. Ninety percent of Hindus in the US are immigrants while 10 percent are converts. In the US, Hinduism has the highest retention rate in comparison to other religions (World Population Review 2022). While determinative figures are hard to pinpoint, Hinduism is likely the third largest religion in the world.

History

The foundation of Hinduism can be traced back to ancient, anonymous Indian sages who claimed to discover eternal truths. These truths are called *apausheya* (not of human invention) as sages realized that these truths had always existed and had come from God (Bhaskarananda 2002: 4; Basham 1998). These sages were called *rishis* (seers) because they had seen or experienced these truths with their purified minds. Hinduism is always evolving, thanks to various sages and saints who have enriched this religion with their teachings. The eternal truths were compiled by sage Vyasa in a book called the *Vedas*. Since then, many different saints, Adi Sankaracharya, Vallabhacharya, and Swami Vivekananda, to name a few, have reformed and revitalized Hinduism and made it relevant to their times. These flexible and evolving characteristics have prompted scholars to describe Hinduism as a way of life rather than a religion.

By the second millennium BCE there was a highly developed civilization in the northwestern part of the south Asian subcontinent called the Indus Valley, which is now a part of Pakistan. Archaeologists have discovered two sites that indicate a high level of social order and planning. These sites are Mohenjo-Daro and Harappa and they once formed a part of a larger social network (Schmidt et al. 1999: 222). By 1500 BCE, a semi-nomadic group called the Aryans invaded this region. The origin of the Aryans is a topic of controversy among scholars. It has been postulated that they may have come from Central Asia (Gafurov 1973: 141, 149), Lithuania (Bender 1922: 55), the Arctic (Tilak 1956: 388–389), or southeastern Europe (Bongard 1980: 123). Some argue that Aryans were indigenous to India (Vivekananda 1947: 293). The Aryans brought with them their gods and their hierarchy of social class. The religious rites of purification and the class system were used to preserve and elevate their race and subjugate the Dravidians, the aboriginals.

The history of religious development in Hinduism is rather complex due to various contributing factors such as the rise of Buddhism, Jainism, Islam, Christianity, and other socio-political developments. Hence it is difficult to place an exact time frame (Radhakrishnan 1956: vol. 2, 22–23). However, the religious development dating back to the arrival of the Aryans in the Indus Valley may be broadly divided into four main periods: the Vedic period (2000–600 BCE), the Ancient period (600 BCE–1000 CE), the Medieval period (1000–1800 CE), and the Modern period (1800–present) (Radhakrishnan 1956: vol. 1, 272).

The Vedic period (2000–600 BCE) represents the earliest developments of the Hindu religion and shows significant theological progression in the understanding of reality and cosmology. There were four major religious and theological texts that this period produced, referred to as *Samhitas, Brahmanas, Aranyakas,* and *Upanishads.*

Samhitas refers to the collection of ancient sayings and consists of four collections of the *Vedas.* The *Rig-Veda* is the earliest *Veda,* dealing with higher gods as conceived by a more advanced class. The *Sama-Veda* is the book of chants. *Yajur-Veda* contains liturgy (including mantras) essential for sacrifices in the religious practice during the Vedic period. Finally, *Atharva-Veda* represents a much more primitive stage of thought in comparison to other *Vedas* (Mark 2020).

The cosmology of this era consisted of the personification of the gods in relation to their historical contexts. There was Mitra, the god of light; Surya, the sun god; Savitr, the god of the solar system; Agni, the god of fire; Soma, the god of breath and inspiration; Varuna, the god of the sky; and Indra, the god of thunder. Gradually, depending on their environmental and historical context, one of the gods became the preferred deity, though other gods were not rejected (henotheism). Indra was essential in matters of war, and Varuna for their agricultural concerns. Varuna was soon given the task of maintaining justice and morality. His role was to watch over the world, punish evil doers, and forgive those who ask for forgiveness. Gradually the concept of *rta* was developed. *Rta* refers to the cosmic order of the universe and the law of righteousness. Varuna, therefore, was the one who implemented the laws of *rta.*

Brahmanas are commentaries on the four *Vedas,* detailing the proper performance of rituals. The *Brahmanas* were seminal in the development of later Hindu thought and scholarship. During the *Samhitas* period, the movement grew from polytheism to henotheism. The *Brahmanas* helped move the developing Hinduism from henotheism to monotheism and from monotheism to monism. The crowding of the gods and goddesses proved to be exhausting to the intellect that seeks pattern and unity. Factors leading to the development of monotheism during this period were the belief in one and only one Supreme Being, unity in this world, and the idea of *rta.* Through these three factors there emerged the understanding of one supreme God. This supreme God was called Visvakarma (maker of the world), sometimes also Prajapati (lord of creatures).

Aranyakas provided the continuity from the *Brahmanas* in the sense that they dealt with the meanings of the "secret" rituals not detailed in the *Brahmanas.* The *Aranyakas* discuss dangerous sacrifices in the style of the *Brahmanas* and thus are primarily concerned with the proper performance of ritual. The *Aranyakas* are "secret" in the sense that they are restricted to a particular class of rituals that were conveyed individually from the teacher to the student.

Still the Hindu mind was not satisfied with deities that embodied human projections. Even the belief in the Supreme Being could not satisfy the search for a unifying principle and the essence of things. This led to the belief that there must be an impersonal ruling force in the universe. "There was then neither non-entity nor entity.... That One breathed calmly, self-supported; then was nothing different from it, or above it" (Muir

1967: 357). This theological development prepared the stage for the next significant religious period, the *Upanishads*.

Upanishads represents one of the most significant religious and philosophical developments during the Vedic period. The term *Upanishads* means to sit nearby or to be mentored by the learned, the sage. *Upanishads*, also called *Vedanta* (the height or culmination of knowledge), represented a very philosophical understanding of life and reality. It aimed at searching for a release from pain and suffering and claimed that attachment to that which is impermanent results in suffering. To escape from suffering, one needs to be attached to that which is permanent. That which is permanent is real. What is that which is permanent? According to *Upanishads*, at the essential core of each of us there is the absolute, constant, permanent, and unchanging bliss called *atman*. And this absolute bliss in each of us is of the same essence as Brahman. Hence the *Upanishads* teaches that *atman* is Brahman. Nothing else is real except Brahman and our attachment to the phenomenal world of change as a result of our ignorance is the primary cause of suffering. According to the *Upanishads*:

> Smaller than the smallest, greater than the greatest, this Self forever dwells within the hearts of all. When a man is free from desire, his mind and senses purified, he beholds the glory of the Self and is without sorrow.
>
> (Prabhavananda & Manchester 1957: 123–124)

The Ancient Period (600 BCE–1000 CE) was an era of myths and narratives and the development of six philosophical systems leading to a more refined approach to *Vedanta* (the union between self and Brahman). The myths and narratives were produced to convey spiritual teachings and lessons. These narratives emerged as a response to challenges by Jainism and Buddhism on the Brahmanic teachings, rituals, and the caste system. A new form of religious literature was needed to provide teachings that could address the masses in a meaningful way. Chief among the stories of this period were the two great Indian epics, *Ramayana* and *Mahabarata*. *Ramayana* tells the story of Rama (the divine incarnation of Vishnu, the god of preservation), who abides by the law of *dharma*, the prescription for ways of conducting oneself within the religious and social realms. Rama portrayed the qualities of an obedient son, a faithful husband, and a responsible ruler. However, because his stepmother wished for her own son to become the ruler of Aydohya instead of Rama, he was banished to the forest for 14 years. His faithful wife, Sita, and his brother, Lakshmana, joined him in the forest. While in the forest, the evil king of Lanka, Ravana, abducted Sita. Rama solicited the help of the monkey king Hanuman, built a bridge to Lanka, and brought Sita safely back to Aydohya. Once they returned to Aydohya, Rama demanded under the pressure of the public that Sita prove her purity before he could receive her back. She did so by walking over a large fire without harm. *Ramayana* describes the ideal way of life exemplified by different characters in the epic, showing the importance of living life according to *dharma*.

Mahabarata tells the story of the conflict and war within a family and the price of abiding by the *dharma*. Within *Mahabarata* is a section called *Bhagavad Gita* (The Song of the Lord), which is one of the most influential sacred texts in Hinduism. In *Bhagavad Gita*, Prince Arjuna of the Pandavas family expresses his anxiety regarding going to battle against his own cousins during a civil war. Lord Krishna, the incarnation of Vishnu, serves as the king's charioteer and while riding into battle taught Arjuna an important lesson on *dharma*. The *Bhagavad Gita* contains 700 verses of dialogue between Krishna and Arjuna regarding the detachment of oneself from the consequence of one's own actions. *Dharma* calls us to act rightly and be willing to accept whatever consequences may come. It is not our duty to attach ourselves to the consequences of our action whether that be positive or negative. We are called to act in accord with *dharma* and that is our sole responsibility. In *Bhagavad Gita*, Lord Krishna instructs Arjuna:

> There are principles to regulate attachment and aversion pertaining to the senses and their objects. One should not come under the control of such attachment and aversion, because they are stumbling blocks on the path of self-realization. It is far better to discharge one's prescribed duties, even though faultily, than another's duties perfectly. Destruction in the course of performing one's own duty is better than engaging in another's duties, for to follow another's path is dangerous.
>
> (Prabhupada 1997: 116–117)

There was also the development of six philosophical systems (*darshanas*) aiming at offering intellectual defence against challenges posted by Jainism and Buddhism. The authors of the six systems wrote treatises using very concise aphorisms called sutras. The first two are *Nyaya* and *Vaisheshika*, which are collections of sutras that provide logic and cosmology, while *Samkhya* offers the basis for the teachings of *Bhagavad Gita*. *Yoga* teaches the discipline of the body as a method of achieving detachment, and *Mimamsa* explores rituals. Finally, *Vedanta* discusses the relationship between the self and Brahman. Within *Vedanta*, there are three major approaches. In *Advaita*, as popularized by Shankara, there is ultimately no distinction between the self and Brahman. The two are one. *Dvaita* of Ramanuja suggests that there is a radical difference between the self and Brahman while *Dvaitadvaita* leaves room for possible tension between these two possibilities (Schmidt et al. 1999: 232–233).

Hindu religious practices during the medieval period (1000–1800 CE) placed emphasis on *bhakti* (devotion). *Bhakti* refers to the belief that liberation through unification between self and Brahman can be achieved through total devotion through singing and chanting often associated with strong emotion and mystical experience with the deity, the type of relationship that is comparable to that between the lover and the beloved (Britannica 2015b). Bhakti as a movement originated from South India and the two main deities were Vishnu (the god who preserves) and Shiva (the god who destroys and recreates). Those who worship Vishnu are called Vaishanavaite and those who worship Shiva are called Shaivite (Hawkins 2004: 49–64).

The Modern period (1800–present) in the development of Hinduism in many ways emerged from an attempt to respond to the influence of Christianity and Western thought. An important development during this era is the religious movement called Brahmo Samaj, founded by Ram Mohan Roy (1772–1833). It was the movement that focused on eliminating discrimination against women, especially that of *sati* (burning of widows along with their deceased husbands), incorporating certain aspects of Christianity, and promoting English-style schools for children. Rabindranath Tagore (the first Indian Nobel laureate) continued the work of Brahmo Samaj and established a Bengali language newspaper and a school for Brahmo Samaj missionaries. Another significant movement during this period came from a Brahmin priest of the Kali temple in Calcutta. Ramakrishna

(1836–1886), who attracted many followers in Calcutta, preached the message of unity of all religions and invited many to renounce worldly possessions and become monks. The teachings of Ramakrishna came to Europe and America through the influential work of one of his followers, Vivekananda (1863–1902), founder of Ramakrishna Mission. He is credited as a major figure in the revival of Hinduism in India (Hawkins 2004: 91–94; Fuller 2010).

Beliefs and practices

General

The practices of Hinduism are based on the beliefs and teachings of the *Vedas*. According to the *Vedas*, there is one Supreme God called Brahman. Other terms used to describe this transcendental God are Absolute Truth, Consciousness, Infinite Bliss, Impersonal God, and Nirguna (attribute-less) Brahman. However, it is very difficult to think of the infinite Brahman with one's finite mind. Thus, the idea of Nirguna Brahman gave way to Saguna Brahman, or Personal God. This Personal God, also known as Ishvara, has three basic aspects: (1) the creator called Brahma, (2) the preserver called Vishnu, and (3) the destroyer called Shiva. These three Gods, Trimurti, form the foundation of beliefs and practices in Hinduism. There are many other aspects of this Personal God, and each of these other aspects can be personified as a deity. The deities are not so much different gods, rather they are the personifications of various aspects of one and the same Ishvara. For example, when Hindus pray for knowledge or learning, they think of Ishvara personified as deity Saraswati (goddess of knowledge). This results in the common misunderstanding that there are many gods in Hinduism. Ultimately, Hinduism asserts one Supreme God and the goal of believers is to merge with this God.

The *Vedas* speaks of the law of eternal duty, or *sanatana dharma*, and refers to the cycle of birth and rebirth (*samsara*) resulting in pain and suffering due to bad deeds (*karma*) and in the path of liberation (*moksha*). These three concepts form the basis for Hindu beliefs and practices. According to the *Vedas*, one's true nature is that of eternal, unchanging self or *atman*. It is to be differentiated from the material and changing self. But through ignorance of the true nature of self, we become attached to this false, physical self, thereby causing a karmic reaction (Basham 1976).

The word karma comes from the root *kri*, which means "to do." Every action becomes karma. These actions are judged and evaluated by the law of causation that states, "You reap what you sow." The concept of karma, derived from *rta*, first appeared in the *Vedas*. *Rta* was the principle that governed both physical and moral actions. During the *Brahmanas* period, it was looked upon as a fixed law of causation applying to all moral conduct. According to this law, every act carries with it an effect. This law does not only apply to this life but extends to the next life as well, associating the doctrine of karma to the doctrine of reincarnation (the cycle of birth and rebirth). The law does not only judge one's external behavior, but also one's intentions behind any given action.

But if a person's life is in accordance with the law of karma, is this person's life pre-determined? Where is the place of freedom? The tension of karma and freedom may be explained on the basis of the three forms of karma. First, *prarabdha* karma may be compared to an arrow that has already been loosed. It refers to fully pre-determined things such as gender, parents, and the color of one's skin. This type of karma is responsible for the pleasures and pains of this present life. Second, *samchita* karma is like an arrow resting in the bow about to be released and refers primarily to character and innate tendencies. It is still possible, in this view of karma, to change one's character and overcome one's tendencies. This change can be achieved by ritualistic acts and through *jnana* (knowledge). *Samchita* karma is accumulated over many past lives and results in good things in future lives. Third, *agami* karma is the arrow that has not yet been placed in the bow. This refers to any action that is performed in this life and may affect results in both this life and the next. *Agami* karma that does not bear any results in this life becomes accumulated as *samchita* karma. Through these various forms of karma, each one of us is the creator and architect of our future. We shape our own life and everything we do has natural consequences.

Samsara, or the cycle of birth and rebirth, is a natural development of the concept of karma. *Samsara* refers to the cycle of birth and rebirth that will continue unceasing as long as karma exists. Karma and *samsara* also help explain the problem of suffering. As long as one is engaged in negative mental, emotional, and behavioral processes, one will remain within this cycle of pain and suffering. The source of rebirth includes the fear of death, the love for the deceased, the illusion regarding the reality of life, and the desire to live. The way out of this suffering is through *moksha*.

The term *moksha* means liberation or emancipation from selfishness, ignorance, and attachment. It is the path that releases one from the cycle of birth and rebirth that causes suffering. The four paths leading to *moksha* are:

1. *Jnana marga* (the path of knowledge). This is the path of liberation through the attainment of right knowledge and understanding. If we do not understand the cause of suffering it would be impossible to be released from *samsara*.
2. *Karma marga* (the path of action). This is the path of liberation through right action, through good deeds that include the correct performance of ritual and sacrifices.
3. *Raj yoga marga* (the path of discipline). The practice of yoga through the discipline of the body and mind can enhance one's concentration on divinity and results in the reduction of bad karma.
4. *Bhakti marga* (the path of devotion). Through devotion of total and fully committed love for God one may achieve liberation (Britannica, 2015a,b).

While life's ultimate goal is to achieve *moksha*, Hindus recognize the importance of various stages of life that one must go through as one matures. First, it is important to practice *dharma*, or good moral conduct, because morality occupies the highest place in Hindu thought. Second, *artha*, or wealth, is an important part of life. A person must work hard to sustain and provide for the family. It is important to remember that earning must be done in an honest manner. The third stage refers to *kama*, worldly desire or pleasure. To acknowledge the realm of passion is to acknowledge the reality of human nature. In Hindu tradition there is nothing wrong with worldly desire as long as it is expressed in appropriate ways. Finally, there is *moksha*. In this final stage the goal is to arrive at *sanyasin*, to be "one who neither hates nor loves anything." This is the stage where one no longer yearns to be "somebody." A *sanyasin* is contented with life and finds harmony within the self. It may be contrasted with the unwise life where one struggles with aging, life, and death (Dimock et al. 2022; Olivelle, 2014).

Health and disease

Health beliefs and practices among Hindus may be dated back to 5000 BCE when sages searched for solutions to the problem of ill health and disease. During the early stage of development, disease was viewed as a punishment from the gods or perturbation of the demons. When transgression took place the god Varuna, who governed moral law, was understood to cause diseases as punishment, while Rudra, the god of ambivalence, inflicted pain at random. According to AL Basham, "Demons as causes of disease loom large in the later collection of hymns known as the Atharva Veda," pointing to the general belief "that illness was caused by evil spirits, who could be expelled by the utterance of the right formula by qualified practitioners, often aided by the administration of herbal remedies and other treatments" (Basham 1976: 19). However, by the sixth or fifth century BCE, the Indian medical system had evolved into its current form. This medical evolution has come to be known as *Ayurveda*, the science of life and longevity about which most Indians possess basic understanding. Ayurvedic medicine is divided into eight categories: (1) general principles of medicine, (2) pathology, (3) diagnosis, (4) physiology and anatomy, (5) prognosis, (6) therapeutics, (7) pharmaceutics, and (8) treatment protocol (Basham 1976: 20). But *Ayurveda* is "not merely a system of medicine"; rather it is "a way of life that aims to increase lifespan by preventing or delaying the aging process. Its objective is to create optimal health and well-being through a comprehensive approach that addresses mind, body, behavior, and environment" (Sharma et al. 2007: 1012). In *Ayurveda*, health is so much more than sickness. Health is a way of living, a way of being that focuses on life-style in alignment with one's philosophy regarding life and reality.

In Ayurvedic terms, health is the balance between body, mind, and spirit. It is about diet and exercise. It consists of the way we see the world. It speaks of the quality of our souls. It believes in positive social relation and perspective in life. It is the perspective that helps reduce stress and encourages balanced living, the type of living that takes time to love, laugh, eat, play, work, and relate to other human beings in a meaningful way. Hence health is not strictly physiological or biological. Health is a perspective in life, one that seeks balance as the primary form of well-being. Restoration of health requires restoration of this balanced perspective in life.

From the perspective of wholeness and balance, the human body consists of three basic elements. These are wind (*vata*), fire (*pitta*), and water (*kapha*). A healthy body results from harmonic balance of these three elements. When any of its elements are out of balance, the system becomes "troubled" (Obeyesekere 1998: 201–202). Desai explains that "an excess of *fire* will produce fever, redness, burning, smells, and discoloration; an excess of *wind* will produce paralysis, cramps, fainting, deafness, and joint pains; and the symptoms of aggravated *moisture* are drowsiness, lethargy, swelling, and stiffness" (Desai 1989: 82). There are two things that may cause such imbalance. External factors include pollution, changing seasons, and infection, and internal factors such as stress, internal conflicts, and grief create imbalance. When the internal is toxic, it weakens the body and hence decreases its ability to fight or resist harmful external factors. The causes for internal toxins are fear, anxiety, anger, greed, sorrow, and envy. The fire element may be aggravated by passion and anger. Sorrow and grief can trouble the moisture, while vanity negatively impacts the wind element (Desai 1989: 82). The build-up of internal toxins can be explained by understanding how blockage within the internal system affects the body. Poor blood circulation resulting from blockage negatively impacts the distribution of nutrition, reduces the flow of oxygen, and results in various physical symptoms such as fatigue, dizziness, and heart palpitation. A journalist, Shubhra Krishan, who spent many years studying Ayurvedic medicine, describes this process:

> On a rushed day, I go on my toxin-collecting spree more systematically. I work late into the night, depriving my body and mind of the rest they need. I wake up irritable and groggy, with little appetite for breakfast. Whatever appetite I have, I douse with three continuous cups of coffee. I go to work and plunge straightaway into the waiting files. I make careless mistakes, then simmer when they're pointed out. Just before a crucial meeting, I find I have gone completely blank. How do these acts of neglect translate into actual toxins? They generate such substance as acid, bile, cholesterol, and adrenaline. In moderate amounts, these are essential to life. But produced in excess, they overwhelm the body, compromising its ability to perform the routine functions of metabolism and digestion normally.
>
> (Krishan 2003: 19–20)

In Ayurvedic terms, these toxins are called *ama*, which means "unripe, immature, undigested" (Krishan 2003: 20). Before we can understand the Ayurvedic approach to cleansing toxins from the body it is important to understand the concept of personal constitution. Each person comes with a core constitution and the constitution emerges from the combination of five basic elements: earth, water, wind, fire, and ether. Because every human being is a microcosm of the universe, these elements are present in each individual. The basic nature of each individual may be divided into three categories: *vata* (ether and air), *pitta* (earth and fire), and *kapha* (water and earth), resulting from various possible combinations of the five elements. Understanding these basic types can help us understand how to restore health and balance.

An individual leaning toward *vata* (wind) tends to be quick in thought and action, and light and thin in build, has dry skin, is sensitive to cold, a light sleeper, tends to worry, and responds positively to warm, cooked foods, and hot beverages. A *pitta* (fire) person has a moderate build, strong appetite and digestion, reddish complexion, is sensitive to hot weather, has a steady memory, can be irritable and quick-tempered, a perfectionistic, and responds well to cold food and beverages. A *kapha* (water) person is normally heavy in build, has great endurance, is slow and methodical, has oily skin, a calm and steady personality, is a heavy sleeper, has slow digestion and mild appetite, and has thick and dark hair (Krishan 2003: 49–51).

Harmonic balance and imbalance may differ from type to type. Factors that cause imbalance in *vata* are: bitter, salty, and astringent tastes, dryness, light, cold foods, late night sleep, excessive exercise, grief, and worry. For *pitta*, imbalance may be caused by pungent, sour, and salty tastes, heat exposure, exhaustion, and anger. *Kapha* persons become imbalanced through sweet, sour, and salty tastes, oily and heavy foods, overeating, lack of exercise, excess sleeping, or napping. Further there are factors that can cause imbalance for all types. These are: eating excessively, improper diet, contaminated food, foul and dry meat, eating food out of season, negative thoughts, and being inactive (Tirtha 1998: 40–41). *Ayurveda* recognizes that different foods, tastes, climates, colors, seasons, and activities affect people differently depending on their basic types. Hence when one recognizes one's type and learns to observe one's responses to diet, environment, seasons, and psychological factors, one may learn to achieve and maintain balance within oneself and thus achieve good health.

As part of the attempt to balance one's health, *Ayurveda* recommends a cleansing process called *panchakarma* (five actions) to get rid of toxins from the body. As the name indicates, this process involves five procedures as follows: (1) vomiting, (2) purgation, (3) enema, (4) elimination of toxins through the nose, and (5) moksha, detoxification of blood.

Hindus approach various health and bioethical issues with a deep reverence for scripture and tradition, though not without sensitivity to modern medicine and technology. On birth control, the *Vedas* do not make a specific prohibition against it, and many modern Hindus practice some form of birth control. As far as abortion is concerned, Hindu scriptures such as the *Rig-Veda, Atharva-Veda*, and *Sushruta Samhita* prohibit abortion, except when the mother's life is in danger. This is primarily because Hinduism is a religion of non-violence. Furthermore, because of the Hindu belief in reincarnation, abortion may be viewed as a negative process that interferes with the cycle of life in accord with one's karma, especially since most Hindus believe that the soul exists at conception. However, attitudes toward elective termination of pregnancy vary among modern Hindus (Coward & Sidhu 2000: 1167–1170; Jootum 2002: 38–40; Coward 2004: 2759–2760).

When considering the issue of diet, most Hindus are lacto-vegetarians and avoid animal products, except milk, in the diet. Even among those who consume animal products, beef and pork are strongly avoided. It is important when working with patients to explain the source of medications, like insulin or pancreatic enzymes, whether or not they come from animal sources. Also, there are certain days of the month and year when fasting is observed in accord with special occasions, mostly related to their personal deities. Fasting is considered to be purifying.

Another issue that needs to be taken into consideration is that of biotechnology. Advances in biotechnology and medical treatments such as stem cell research have further complicated Hindus' approach to healthcare and ethics. There are no historical examples of such innovations in scripture, making present-day recommendations difficult. However, there are various governmental agencies in India, such as the Department of Biotechnology and the Indian Council of Medical Research, that help provide answers to the moral and ethical questions arising from the use of biotechnology (Jayaraman 1997: 838; Mudur 2001: 530).

Death and dying

Hindus believe the body is a vehicle for the soul or *atman* through which it can experience the world and progress on its journey to God. At the time of death, this body is discarded and *atman* takes on another body; this cycle of changing bodies continues until *atman* reaches its final goal – union with God. Hindus believe that *atman* is immortal, while the physical body is perishable. They believe that suffering at the time of death is due to karma and therefore inevitable. Many prefer to die at home and may want to have specific ritual or religious rites performed. Many prefer to listen to sacred chants from scriptures and have drops of sacred water from the Ganges River put in their mouth at the time of death. A dying person may wish to be moved to the floor to be close to Mother Earth. After death, close family members wash the body, a priest may perform religious rites, and then the body is cremated, preferably within 24 hours. Children younger than 3 years of age, however, are usually simply buried. There is a 10–14-day period of family mourning. Since death is seen as a period of transition into the next life, excessive mourning is discouraged. During this period of mourning, family members do not perform religious ceremonies. They eat simple vegetarian food and wear white clothing as a symbol of mourning. At the end of the mourning period, a religious ceremony is performed to ensure that the deceased has a peaceful transition to the next life. It is beneficial to understand possible beliefs and ritual practices that may occur such as the drinking of holy water from the Ganges, placing Tulsi leaf on the tongue, embracing physical pain (help reduce negative karma), placing the head of the body toward the north and toes to the south, pictures of patient's deity, chanting holy verses and lighting a candle (Chandratre & Soman, 2022).

Suicide is perceived as a bad way to die and a reprehensible act. Similarly, euthanasia is discouraged. Artificial life support is not viewed favorably as most Hindus believe that prolonging life after a person's time for death interferes with karma and disrupts the cycle of reincarnation. Organ donation and transplants are acceptable and not subject to the same laws on non-violence, since the donors chose to give of themselves out of their own free will (unlike animals). Some Hindus, however, disagree as they believe every action has karmic implications and something as serious as replacing a major organ can carry

Table 5.1 Dos and don'ts

Dos	Don'ts
1. Be aware of philosophical reasons for particular behaviors or decisions in medical care.	1. Do not remove jewelry, adornments, or threads without discussing with the patient as they have religious significance.
2. Recognize that fasting is a common practice and may affect medical/dietary plans.	2. Do not disregard family members when making medical decisions.
3. Be sensitive to concerns about modesty.	3. Do not use left hand (if possible) when performing tasks on the patients (due to cultural understanding of cleanliness) and be cautious when handling patient's hand movement in any way (starting an intravenous line etc.).
4. Discuss possibility of imminent death with family members regarding location or religious rituals and rites.	
5. Provide caregivers of the same sex.	4. Do not disregard times for prayer or meditation and avoid medical procedures or examinations during those times.
6. Understand that strong belief in astrology may prevent a family from naming a newborn before leaving the hospital or agreeing to a certain time for elective surgery.	
7. Understand that pain and suffering may be seen as the result of karma and may impact the patient's self-report of pain.	5. Do not disregard dietary preference and patients' hesitation to use medications with animal by-products.
8. Take into account ideas about "hot" and "cold" food theory in Ayurvedic thought.	6. Do not touch Hindu scriptures with feet or put them on the floor as to do so would be a grave insult.
9. Remove shoes before entering the Hindu home (home of healthcare workers).	
10. Note the exact time of birth.	

some of the donor's karma to the recipient. Additionally, some believe that since a part of the deceased donor's physical body still "lives" this may interfere with the donor's soul moving on to the next incarnation.

Conclusion

Hinduism is a complex religion that accommodates wide variation of beliefs and practices in relation to conceptual understanding of deities and related rituals and rites. However, within these wide variations we find common themes permeating the world of Hindu religious beliefs – the path leading to oneness with Brahman, the Ultimate Reality, as a symbol of eternal bliss, and the practice of non-violence. In relation to health, religion plays a significant role in showing the connection between physical well-being and Hindu cosmology. By pursuing optimal health through the balance of body, mind, and spirit, Hindus seek to experience wholeness in this life and build positive karma for the lives to come – until they ultimately reach *moksha*.

Case study #1

Hindus use cremation as a central feature of their last rites. Traditionally these crema-tion ceremonies take place near the bank of a river using wood to burn the bodies. The holiest place for cremation ceremonies is on the bank of the Ganges River in India where cremations happen day and night. As part of the ritual, ashes are collected and scattered into the river. This ritual practice is increasing the levels of pollution in the river all across India but particularly in the Ganges River and riverbanks.

There are broad environmental concerns. Twenty-seven thousand Indians die each day with most bodies cremated. Around 650 pounds of wood are needed to burn each body. As a result, "The ashes of millions of dead have turned the water into a stinking, polluted swirl. Worse, since wood is expensive, bodies sometimes are thrown into the river half-burned," according to *Associated Press* correspondent, Nirmala George (2003). There is also the environment impact from consuming so much wood to perform the ritual resulting in denuded forests. Hindu scholars have declared that cremation with wood on the bank of the Ganges is not a central teaching of Hinduism though it remains a long-standing tradition. More efficient electric furnaces that cost less and produce smaller amounts of ash are provided by the Indian government. But most grieving relatives con-tinue to insist on the traditional practice.

The care and disposal of the dead is a sacred responsibility of the living in most religions. In this case, however, such traditions may also be creating a public health risk as well.

Questions for reflection

1. Given the environmental damage and the public health risks, should public health officials take the initiative to limit or even prohibit this practice of ritual burning on riverbanks?
2. How can public health officials work with religious leaders to reduce the environment impact of Hindu's burial rituals? How might religious thought leaders change public opinion?

3. Some religions forbid cremation, including Islam and Orthodox Judaism. Along with Hindus, most Buddhists and Sikhs practice cremation. What beliefs about the afterlife might account for the differences?

*Submitted by Andy Lampkin

Case study #2

A Hindu male in his early 40s came to a small, rural critical access hospital. The patient was experiencing abdominal pain, constipation, and flatulence and was admitted for further observation.

When the unit nurse came to see him, the patient was kneeling over a trash can, vomiting, and expressed a desperate need to use the restroom. The nurse helped him to the restroom. The nurse thought these were additional symptoms that might indicate what was going on with the patient's GI tract, so she informed his physician.

Entering his room, now with the doctor, they saw what looked like laxatives and a vial with unidentified organic content of an ipecac-like substance on the heat register in his room next to his backpack. The doctor and nurse presumed correctly that they were intended for purging. The patient explained that he had begun taking the initial steps of *Ayurveda* cleansing.

The doctor wondered why the patient thought this purging was a good idea and why, given the pain he was in, he had brought them with him to the hospital. The patient discontinued the purging and remained in the hospital for observation and hydration for 48 hours.

Questions for reflection

1. What do you know about *Ayurveda* cleansing (panchakarma), including therapeutic purging (verechana)? How might you learn more about this patient's practice and the substances he ingested?
2. How can this patient's medical team respect his spiritual/religious practices while also providing him with the best medical care?
3. Ayurveda medicine is a vast field of knowledge and practice largely unknown in the West. What would be the possible benefits and drawbacks in including an introduction to Ayurveda theory and practice in conventional Western medical education?

*Submitted by Garrett Potts

Glossary

Atman The true self that transcends the phenomenal world of our daily existence.
Ayurveda This term means the science of life and refers to the system of traditional medicine native to India.
Bhagavad Gita One of the sacred scriptures in Hinduism containing 700 verses of conversation between Krishna and Arjuna regarding the path toward self-realization. It also forms a part of the larger text, the *Mahabarata*.
Brahman The Divine ground of all reality that is unchanging, infinite, unconditional, and immanent.

Dharma The path leading to righteous living.

Karma An action or deed governed by the law of causality that can result in positive or negative direction in future lives and in the cycle of birth and rebirth.

Moksha This equates with salvation, the final liberation from the cycle of birth and rebirth, resulting in union with Brahman.

Samsara The cycle of birth and rebirth.

Vedas The term Vedas means "knowledge" and refers to the oldest compilation of sacred scriptures in the Hindu tradition.

Note

1 Manoj Shah, one of the original authors of this chapter, was unable to be involved in the update for this third edition.

Bibliography

Basham, AL. (1976) "The Practice of Medicine in Ancient and Medieval India," in Leslie, C. (ed.) *Asian Medical Systems: A Comparative Study* (pp. 18–43). Berkeley, CA: University of California Press.

Bender, HH. (1922) *The Home of the Indo-Europeans.* New Jersey: Princeton University Press.

Bhagavad Gita, The (2007) (E. Easwaran, Trans.) 2nd ed. California: Nilgiri Press.

Bhaskarananda, S. (2002) *The Essentials of Hinduism: A Comprehensive Overview of the World's Oldest Religion.* Seattle, WA: Viveka Press.

Bongard, GM. (1980) *The Origin of the Aryans.* Delhi, India: Arnold-Heinemann.

Britannica, Encyclopedia of (2015) "Marga." www.britannica.com/topic/marga-Indian-religion

Britannica, Encyclopedia of (2015b) "Bhakti." www.britannica.com/topic/bhakti

Chandratre, S., and Soman, A. (2022) "End of Life Care Practices for Hindu Patients During COVID-19," *Journal of Palliative Care,* 37(1): 3–7. https://doi.org/10.1177/0825859721 1036243

Coward, H. (2004) "Hindu Bioethics for the Twenty-First Century," *Journal of the American Medical Association, 291(22):* 2759–2760.

Coward, H., and Sidhu, T. (2000) "Bioethics for Clinicians: Hinduism and Sikhism," *Canadian Medical Association Journal, 163(9):* 1167–1170.

Desai, P. (1989) *Health and Medicine in the Hindu Tradition.* New York: Crossroad.

Dimock, EC., Narayanan, V., Smith, BK., Basham, AL., Buitenen, JAB., van Doniger, W., and Gold, AG. (2022) "Hinduism," *Encyclopedia Britannica.* www.britannica.com/topic/Hinduism

Fuller, J. (2010) "Teaching Modern Hinduism," *Teaching About Asian Religions, 15(2).* www.asianstudies.org/publications/eaa/archives/teaching-modern-hinduism/

Gafurov, BG. (1973) *From Ancient History to Contemporary Times Central Asia.* Delhi, India: Navyug.

George, N. (2003) "India's Burial Rites Put Nature at Risk," Associated Press. August 17, 2003. www.washingtonpost.com/archive/politics/2003/08/17/indias-burial-rites-put-nature-at-risk/404ee316-5ec5-4e28-849a-4adf512a852e/

Hawkins, B. (2004) *Asian Religions.* New York: Pearson/Longman.

Jayaraman, KS. (1997) "India May Set Up Genetics Advisory Panel," *Nature, 387:* 838.

Jootum, D. (2002) "Nursing with Dignity – Part 7: Hinduism," *Nursing Times, 98(15):* 38–40.

Krishan, S. (2003) *Essential Ayurveda: What It Is & What It Can Do for You.* Novato, CA: New World Library.

Mark, JJ. (2020) "The Vedas," *World History Encyclopedia.* www.worldhistory.org/The_Vedas/

Mudur, G. (2001) "India to Tighten Rules of Human Embryonic Stem Cell Research," *British Medical Journal, 2001(323):* 530.

Muir, J. (1967) *Original Sanskrit Texts*, 2nd ed. Amsterdam: Oriental Press.

Obeyesekere, G. (1976) "The Impact of Ayurvedic Ideas on the Culture and the Individual in Sri Lanka," in Leslie, C. (ed.) *Asian Medical Systems: A Comparative Study* (pp. 201–226). Berkeley, CA: University of California Press.

Olivelle, P. (2014) "Moksha," *Encyclopedia Britannica*. www.britannica.com/topic/moksha-Indian-religion

Prabhavananda, S., and Manchester, F. (Trans.) (1957) *The Upanishads: Breath of the Eternal*. New York: Mentor Books.

Prabhupada, AC. (1997) *Bhagavat-Gita as It Is*. Los Angeles: Bhaktivendata.

Radhakrishnan, S. (1956) *Indian Philosophy*, vols 1 and 2. Bombay: Blackie & Son.

Schmidt, R., Sager, G., Carney, G., Jackson, Jr., J., Muller, A., and Zanca, K. (1999) *Patterns of Religion*. Belmont, CA: Wadsworth Publishing.

Sharma, H., Chandola, HM., Singh, G., and Basisht, G. (2007) "Utilization of Ayurveda in Health Care: An Approach for Prevention, Health Promotion, and Treatment of Disease; Part 1 – Ayurveda, the Science of Life," *The Journal of Alternative and Complementary Medicine*, 13(9): 1012.

Tilak, BG. (1956) *The Arctic Home in Vedas*. Pune, India: Tilak Brothers.

Tirtha, SS. (1998) *The Ayurveda Encyclopedia: Natural Secrets to Healing, Prevention, & Longevity*. Bayville, NY: Ayurveda Holistic Center Press.

Vivekananda, S. (1947) *The Complete Works of Swami Vivekananda*, vol. 3. Calcutta, India: Vedanta Press.

World Population Review (2022) Hindu Countries 2022. https://worldpopulationreview.com/country-rankings/hindu-countries

Young, W. (2005) *The World's Religions: Worldviews and Contemporary Issues*. New Jersey: Prentice Hall.

6 Buddhism

Siroj Sorajjakool and Supaporn Naewbood[1]

As rain breaks through a poorly thatched house, passion will break through an unreflecting mind. As rain does not break through a well-thatched house, passion will not break through a well-reflecting mind.

(Dammapada n.d. 1:13–14)

Introduction

Pain is often the reason that makes us ponder the deep meaning of life. It propels us toward this difficult quest until we discover the answer. But for a person to live in the presence of prosperity and comfort while determining to find the answer to this perplexing question, one has to be destined for this task. This was the life of Gautama, the man who, although born into wealth and royalty, abandoned all in the quest for the solution to the question of suffering. Why suffering and what is the path that leads to the cessation of suffering?

Demographics

There are approximately 506 million Buddhists globally representing 6.6 percent of the world population making Buddhism the fourth largest religion (World Population Review 2022). The followers of Buddhism may be divided into three main schools of thought: Theravada Buddhism consists of 38 percent of the total Buddhist population (Nepal, India, Sri Lanka, Thailand, Myanmar, and Cambodia), 56 percent embraces Mahayana Buddhism (China, Japan, Korea, Taiwan, Vietnam, and Singapore), and 6 percent belongs to Tantric Buddhism (Tibet and parts of India) (Buddha Dharma Association and BuddhaNet n.d.). According to World Population Review on religious identity, there are 4.2 million Buddhists in the United States, which is approximately 1.2 percent of the total population (World Population Review 2022).

History

Siddharta Gautama was born around 565 BCE to the Shakya clan in Lumbini (which is now Nepal). His father was Suddhodana, the ruler of Kapilavastu, and his mother, Maya. The story is told that Maya had a night vision in which she saw a white elephant (symbolizing holiness) entering into her body. Nine months later she gave birth to Gautama in a garden in Lumbini. The day he was born, he walked seven steps and in the place where

DOI: 10.4324/9781003288862-6

his footsteps fell lotus flowers blossomed. Seven days later his mother passed away. Not long after his birth, sage Asita announced to the king that the young prince would either become a great king or a great holy man. The sage's message persuaded Suddhodana to shield his son from any religious teachings and human tragedy. Under such a protective environment, Gautama grew up, married Yasodara, and had a son.

It seems, however, that nothing could prevent Gautama from the destiny to which he was called. Even in his comfortable life, he witnessed three human conditions that changed the entire course of his life. He saw sickness, old age, and death. And while pondering this human predicament, he came across an ascetic (someone exercising rigorous, severe self-discipline and self-denial). The image of this ascetic convinced him of his calling. In the middle of the night he left Yasodara and his son, Rahula. Discarding his robe and cutting his hair as a symbol of his decision to give up the life of abundance, he abandoned the palace in search of truth and liberation from pain and suffering.

For six years Gautama went through various forms of intense quest for liberation. He first attempted the Brahmanic meditative approach as taught in the Upanishads (Hindu sacred text). When that did not work, he committed himself to extreme asceticism where he wandered naked throughout the countryside, fasted continually, and often spent sleepless nights searching for truth. During this period five other ascetics joined him. Gautama realized that these ascetic practices only led to physical deterioration and not spiritual enlightenment. He came to the conclusion that both extremes (pleasure and self-denial) would not be beneficial spiritually and decided to take the middle path. In the region called Bodh Gaya, he sat under a bodhi tree and told himself that he would remain there until he discovered the truth about suffering and the path toward liberation. Sitting in a meditative position, Gautama was tempted by Mara, the Hindu god of desire, calling him to return to his life of pleasure and luxury. Firm in his commitment, Gautama continued his quest with his right hand pointing toward the earth (symbolizing the earth as his witness). While meditating under this bodhi tree he "awakened" from the slumber of worldly delusions and understood the cause and the way out of suffering. He became the enlightened Buddha. His emphasis on the "middle path" attracted many followers in India who were searching for liberation but found the esoteric teachings of the Upanishads difficult to achieve. He continued to proclaim his message and laid the foundation of the Buddhist order of monks for the next 45 years.

In 250 BCE a great division occurred among the leadership in Buddhism regarding enlightenment. Those who believed that enlightenment was for all called themselves Mahayana (the great vehicle or big vessel), while the other group was known as Hinayana (the small vehicle). Because of the negative connotation, the Hinayana group began to call themselves Theravada (the Way of the Elders).

Theravada Buddhism is found mostly in India, Sri Lanka, Myanmar, Laos, Thailand, and Cambodia. According to Theravada Buddhism, the Buddha possessed many human qualities and was not insulated from making mistakes. The ethical teachings of Theravada Buddhism are to abstain from evil and the accumulation of material goods, purify one's mind through meditation, and gain right understanding through the Four Noble Truths. Philosophically, Theravada Buddhism emphasizes that Nirvana is a state free from passion, ill will, and delusion. It is a state beyond description. An *arahat* is a person who arrives at this stage and therefore is able to end the cycle of birth and rebirth.

Mahayana Buddhism may be translated as the big vessel because it offers greater possibility for the attainment of liberation than does Theravada Buddhism. Mahayana Buddhism is commonly practiced in China, Japan, Taiwan, Korea, Singapore, and Vietnam. Among the more popular Mahayana schools are Zen, Pure Land, and Tantric Buddhism. Mahayana emphasizes meditation as an attempt to attain the state of quiescence. Its aim is to empty oneself and attain the transcendental state of mind. The Mahayana School believes that the Buddha is no longer the historical sage of the Sakyas clan but he is supra-mundane (above physical manifestation). Mahayana Buddhism teaches the concept of *Bodhicitta* or the awakening of consciousness emphasizing liberation through recognizing *sunyata* (emptiness). *Sunyata* shows us that our incessant, mundane attachments only entrap us within the cycle of pain and suffering. Through meditation one may be awakened and find liberation. The concept of *Boddhisatva* is also one of the main foci. This concept teaches that the goal of life is to be enlightened but that one must forgo entrance to Nirvana in order to assist other creatures through compassion and wisdom, helping them discover the path for the cessation of suffering.

In India around 272 BCE King Ashoka's empire extended from southeast of the Caspian Sea to the Indus valley. At the end of the eight years of his reign, he invaded the country of Kalinga (Orissa), India. During this invasion many thousands died. Upon seeing the effect of war, King Ashoka was struck with sorrow and grief, which led him to embrace Buddhism and he adopted non-violence as the state policy. From his desire to spread this message, he sent representatives to Syria, Egypt, and Greece. His son Mahinda and his sister Samghamata went to Sri Lanka, which became a stronghold of Theravadins from that time on, while his other son, Kantana, took the message to the northwest of India. Theravada Buddhism continued to spread to Burma, Thailand, Cambodia, and Laos.

Theravada Buddhism was introduced to China during the first century CE, but the growth was slow. The emphasis on monasticism did not go well with the traditional concept of ancestor worship that promoted marriage and family. When Mahayana Buddhism was later introduced, the Chinese responded positively because the concept of heavenly beings in Mahayana could accommodate ancestor worship and sons who became Buddhists could continue to help their ancestors. Since that time, Mahayana Buddhism has continued to grow and spread to Japan, Tibet, Central Asia, Taiwan, Vietnam, and Korea (Matthews 1999: 149).

While it is believed that Buddhism was in conversation with the Western world as early as the first century CE, it became much more visible in the nineteenth century due to immigrants from China and Japan and later from Southeast Asia to Europe and the US. Many temples were established for members to engage in religious ceremonies and rituals. During the 1960s, when young people were searching for new experiences, a significant growth in Buddhism took place. Important Buddhist figures in the West included DT Suzuki (1870–1966), who popularized Zen in the West, Thich Nhat Hanh (1926–2022), a popular Vietnamese monk, and the Dalai Lama from Tibet. Today there is a rapid increase of Buddhist communities in the US and Canada through Buddhists who immigrated from Asian countries and indigenous converts. Since the mid twentieth century, the establishment of meditation centers in the US and Canada has been rising as more people turn toward meditation and mindfulness to deal with stressors and enhance their spirituality (Reynolds et al. 2023).

Three branches of Buddhism

There are mainly three branches of Buddhism. These are Theravada Buddhism, Mahayana Buddhism, and Vajrayana Buddhism. Theravada is prominent in South and Southeast Asia regions such as Sri Lanka, Myanmar, Thailand, and Laos. Mahayana Buddhism is commonly practiced in China, Korea, Vietnam, and Japan, while Vajrayana is found mainly in Tibet and Nepal. While there are variations to these branches, they share some common core beliefs in the teaching of the Buddha including the Four Noble Truths.

Theravada is also known as the way of the elders. It is theologically more conservative and focuses on the way to end suffering. It claims to be the original form of Buddhism and the path toward detachment is through meditation and monastic practices. The path toward enlightenment is more individualistic rather than collective. In Theravada, it takes countless cycles of birth and rebirth to achieve true enlightenment.

Mahayana Buddhism focuses on the concept of Bodhicitta or the awakened heart where followers aim to discover the Buddha within while practicing *metta* and *karuna* (love and kindness). It is in the discovery of the Buddha within that provides the way out of suffering. This concept differs significantly from Theravada whose teachings focus on the historical Buddha. The concept of Bodhicitta, because of its wider application, is available to a greater number of people. In Theravada Buddhism, only through monkhood is enlightenment achieved. Whereas in Mahayana, the laity, through diligent practices, can become enlightened as well. Mahayana also believe in deterring entering to Nirvana for the sake of others. They are committed to helping others achieve Nirvana through continual rebirths until all find enlightenment.

Vajrayana, the last branch of Buddhism, is also known as the diamond vehicle or the esoteric path. It shares significant similarities with Mahayana Buddhism. Vajrayana focuses on rituals and symbols as the means toward enlightenment. Vajrayana also believe that through practice of prescribed rituals, it is possible to achieve enlightenment in a single life-time. This is due to the central conception in Vajrayana. While Theravada believes in letting go of all attachment and Mahayana on the possibility of enjoyment in life while pursuing enlightenment, Vajrayana does not promote suppressing attachment but focuses on recognizing and transforming this energy into something positive. In order to harness this energy, Vajrayana emphasizes recitation of *mantra*, practices of certain hand gestures, and paying attention to *mandala* (diagrams of deities and divinity) (Mark 2020).

Beliefs and practices

General

It was in the Deer Park in Benares, a city located by the bank of the Ganges River in India, that the Buddha gave his first sermon on the cause and cessation of suffering, now known as "The Four Noble Truths and the Eightfold Path":

> And this, monks, is the noble truth of the origination of stress: the craving that makes for further becoming — accompanied by passion & delight, relishing now here & now there — i.e., craving for sensual pleasure, craving for becoming, craving for non-becoming.

And this, monks, is the noble truth of the cessation of stress: the remainderless fading & cessation, renunciation, relinquishment, release, & letting go of that very craving.

(*Dhammacakkappavattana Sutta* 1993: para 6,7)

The Buddha teaches that the way out of suffering is through the practice of the Eight Noble Paths. However, common among lay Buddhists is the practice of the Five Precepts that call for abstention from five types of activities: (1) taking life; (2) taking what is not given; (3) sexual immorality; (4) false speech; and (5) intoxication. A more devout Buddhist may seek to practice the Eight Precepts, which include abstention from three additional acts: (1) eating at a wrong time (eat only one meal per day after sunrise and before noon); (2) entertainment and self-adornment such as music, dancing, and jewelry and other types of ornamentation; and (3) luxury and extravagance of all types. It is not uncommon for lay Buddhists to keep the Eight Precepts during the three-month-long Buddhist Lent Day (beginning on the full moon of the eighth lunar month believed to be the day Buddha preached his first sermon).

The teachings of the Buddha may be summarized in three main concepts. These are the belief that life consists of suffering and suffering exists because there is nothing permanent in life, including the self. When one comes to understand that there is no real self, one will find liberation from suffering.

Suffering (dukkha)

"To be is to suffer" is the essential Buddhist assessment of the human existential situation. We are, therefore we suffer. The Buddha taught that birth is painful, decay is painful, disease is painful, death is painful, union with the unpleasant is painful, separation from the pleasant is painful, and unsatisfied cravings are also painful. When we are attached, we set ourselves up for suffering. When we are attached to life, death is painful. When we are attached to others, their departure becomes unbearable. What feeds this attachment is our thirst or our cravings (*tanha*). Buddha teaches that it is the craving desire that leads to becoming. The process of becoming results in the formation of bodily senses (sight, sound, smell, taste, and feeling) leading to gratification. *Tanha* is the fundamental problem of human suffering. It is desire that exacerbates the pain. Most pain we experience in our day-to-day living can be traced back to *tanha*. Desire and attachment are not bad in and of themselves, but only in relation to the second fundamental truth in Buddhism, impermanence. If our attachment is to that which is permanent, lasting happiness could be conceivable. However, what we desire is always in a state of flux: changing and reconfiguring. If we are attached to something we like and that which we really like remains with us all the time, we may not experience suffering. Unfortunately, this is not the case. To answer this tormenting question pertaining to the certainty of life and of the things we desire, the Buddha points us to the doctrine of *anicca* or impermanence.

Impermanence (anicca)

"Then, bhikkhus, it occurred to me: 'The pleasure and joy that arise in dependence on form: this is the gratification in form. That form is impermanent, suffering, and subject to change: this is the danger in form'" (*Samyuta Nikaya* 2000: 22:28). Things we want never remain the same. Life comes and goes. Youth turns to old age. Beauty becomes blemish. Memories deteriorate. Things decay. Nothing is permanent and that is why attachment to such things becomes painful. A river may appear the same, but is it the same river? Contents of the stream, rocks, sand, and pebbles continue to change and reconfigure themselves. Every person goes through the process of continual changes. At every moment we are not the same and yet not the other. We are not the same because our constituent elements change at every moment. Further events that happen in our lives and the information we receive every day are reminders that who we are today are not quite the same as yesterday. At the same time, we are not the other because what we are is the result of our past karma (action). Although the appearances of the world and the "I" seem permanent, a careful analysis shows that nature truly is continually changing. All things are operated by the law of causality. A thing is only a state of which the first is said to be the cause of the second because every action has its consequence. Existence is only a continuity of changes, each of which is determined by its pre-existing conditions. Nothing exists without a condition, and if there is a condition for its existence dissolution is inevitable.

A soul that seeks deliverance must grasp the truth that encompasses the whole of existence – life is *anicca*. And this includes human beings. There is no being in *anicca*, rather there is only becoming which is conditioned by the law of causality. Therefore, everything will inevitably end in dissolution. So, the Buddha teaches that if our ignorance regarding the world as being permanent leads to attachment and thus suffering, the reverse process, the knowledge of all things being impermanent, can lead to detachment and thus liberation.

No-self (anatta)

The doctrine of *anatta* is the belief that behind the phenomenon we call "self" there is no real self. There is no real "I." What I come to claim as myself is but an illusion caused by the desire to become and to be. The concept of "self" is a perplexing one. What is this self? When we move from one social context to another, we could possibly feel and think very differently about ourselves. Further, is it possible that we would perceive ourselves very differently if we were raised in a different place, culture, or socio-economic setting? So, who is this being identified by my name?

The Buddha teaches that the illusion that there is a real self is the primary cause for attachment that results in suffering. If there is no real self, there is no need to be attached, and when there is no attachment, there is no suffering. This self is nothing but an integration of the four elements (aggregates): earth, water, wind, and fire. Every integration implies the possibility of disintegration. Hence this self is impermanent. It is nothing but a combination of the four basic elements that come together based on the law of karma, the law of cause of effect. In explaining the process of becoming or acquiring the illusion of this self, the Buddha points us to the law of *paticcasamuppada*, or the law of dependent origination, the doctrine that seeks to explain how physical and psychological phenomena are conditionally related to each other. The following are constituent parts of the law of *paticcasamuppada*:

1. Ignorance (*avijja*): Through ignorance arises karma formation. Karma formation can be either unwholesome or wholesome. Unwholesome karma formation refers to one's ignorance that may lead to craving (*tanha*), which results in bad deeds. Wholesome karma formation refers to action based on the right understanding.
2. Karma formation (*sankhara*): Through karma formation arises consciousness.
3. Corporeality and mentality (*nama-rupa*): Through consciousness arise corporeality and mentality, or the physical and the mental aspect of a human being.
4. Six bases (*salayatanam*): Through corporeality and mentality arise six bases. These six bases are: eyes, ears, nose, tongue, body, and mind. They provide contact with the external world.
5. Impression (*phasso*): Through the six bases arise impression. Impression is produced when senses come in contact with the objects of attention.
6. Feeling (*vedana*): Through impression arises feeling. Feeling arises as an immediate concomitance of impression.
7. Craving (*tanha*): Through feeling arises craving. The craving to be detached from that which is unpleasant or be united with that which is pleasant arises from the illusion of the self and the world.
8. Clinging (*upadanam*): Through craving arises clinging.
9. Becoming (*bhavo*): Through clinging arises becoming.
10. Rebirth (*jati*): Through becoming arises rebirth.
11. Old age and death (*jutipaccaya jara-maranam*): Through rebirth arises old age and death, thus suffering.

This doctrine of *paticcasamuppada* helps us realize that in the final analysis there is no self. To understand *anatta* is to know the path leading to the cessation of suffering.

Health and disease

Health is an important aspect in the practice of Buddhism. Understanding the Buddhist concept of health requires an understanding of the Buddhist views of pain, suffering, and enlightenment. Buddhism approaches health from a holistic perspective. Health is the harmonious balance of the body, mind, emotion, and the spiritual dimension, and therefore is not merely the absence of disease. What brings about this harmony is the right understanding of the teachings of Buddha. Hence Buddhist understanding of health is closely connected to spirituality (Wijesinghe 2013; Wiist et al. 2012). "According to Buddhism, to be active and healthy, one needs to live a spiritual life" (Hewapathirane 2004: 6). Spirituality is essential because good health derives primarily from correct understanding of the meaning of life and from right practices in accord with the teachings of Buddhism. It requires that one realizes the goal of life, the attainment of enlightenment, through cultivating right understanding, practicing meditation, exerting moderation, and offering compassion. Disease, on the other hand, is the result of ignorance leading to craving desire, impurity, and indulgence that leads to disharmony at the physical, emotional, and spiritual levels. This approach to health points to a strong connection between mind and body. In explaining this relationship, Pinit Ratanakul (2004), professor of religious studies at Mahidol University, affirms that in Buddhism no one can harm us except ourselves. Our thoughts dictate our happiness and through it we can either degrade or improve our well-being.

Recent studies on meditation have affirmed the importance of this aspect of Buddhist teaching pertaining to health practice. In 2001, Richard Davidson and Jon Kabat-Zin carried out a study on meditation with a Tibetan Buddhist monk by placing hundreds of sensors on the monk and connecting them to an EEG, a brain-scanning device. When the monk meditated on compassion, the sensors registered a dramatic shift to a state of great joy. Other studies also reveal the positive impact meditation has on the immune system, blood pressure, depression, and stress (Hewapathirane 2004: 7). A study by Somporn Kantharadussadee-Triamchaisri and associates (2004) on the practice of Buddhism among AIDS patients in Thailand shows that Buddhists who practice positive thinking, contentment, compassion, and meditation show significant decreases in their cortisol and stress levels.

This holistic understanding of health does not preclude the utilization of Western medicine. Buddhism promotes every possible means for good health. However, it is important that "disease" is not viewed merely as physical symptoms. As such another fundamental concept contributing to the understanding of health has to be taken into consideration.

While Western medicine treats the body, it lacks the understanding of the way in which one's karma impacts one's health, causing various forms of disease. According to Ratanakul, "Buddhism attributes karma as an important contributing factor to health and disease. In the Buddhist perspective good health is the correlated effect of good karma in the past and vice versa" (Ratanakul 2004: 162). In explaining the role of karma, Ratanakul points to cases of patients who failed to thrive even when the treatment was successful and those who survived even when their medical care was poor. "Karma is created by choices we made in past lives. Health is to be gained by continuing personal efforts in this life. Good deeds lead to good health whereas bad deeds in this and previous lives bring illness" (Ratanakul 2004: 163). While Buddhism recognizes the place of karma in sickness and disease, it is advised that patients do not use this as an excuse for not taking care of their health but to take advantage of every possible means for healing while being mindful of the Buddhist view of life. Because of the emphasis on the mind–body connection, a healthy body plays a significant role in the path toward enlightenment. Through this understanding of the role of karma, it is important that patients learn to accept the reality of disease in their lives and at the same time make positive efforts to comply with medical advice while working on positive karmic formation that will contribute to their overall health and well-being in this life and the life to come.

In Buddhism, karma is not viewed strictly on the individual basis. There is also a collective dimension of karma and this may refer to the environmental and social factors that can aggravate or mitigate an individual's health and well-being, such as unhealthy or dangerous working conditions. In viewing this collective dimension of karma, it is necessary that governmental agencies play an appropriate role in monitoring and managing healthcare systems and work environments (Ratanakul 2004: 163).

When viewing karma from the context of terminal illness, it becomes even more essential to address the spiritual dimension by promoting cultivation of right understanding, mindfulness, and right practice that will generate positive karma to promote well-being, both for the current state and for life to come.

There are a couple of important considerations we need to pay attention to when treating Buddhist patients, such as the issues of diet and the Buddhist's view of abortion. There is generally no restriction when it comes to diet for Buddhists. While vegetarianism is encouraged among all Buddhists, most in the Theravada tradition do not practice vegetarianism. However, a strict Mahayana Buddhist will avoid eating fish and meat. Buddhists who worship *Guan Yin* (the goddess of mercy) do not eat beef. Some Buddhists avoid eating food prepared with onions and garlic due to the belief that they arouse the base senses. Generally, Buddhists practice moderation when it comes to food and avoid intoxication since it is forbidden by one of the Five Precepts.

When the conception of self begins and ends is occasionally a point of contention in Buddhism. Abortion is an issue in Buddhism because of the reality of this contention. Like other specific issues, abortion is best understood within the broad religious perspective on suffering and the cessation of suffering within life's cycle such as birth, sickness, and death. Life's ultimate goal is the end of suffering which comes when one is no longer caught within the cycle of birth and death. One's birth is determined by one's previous karma (the merits or the lack thereof from one's past life). This fundamental belief forms the basis for the Buddhist approach to ethical issues such as abortion and end-of-life care, including such issues as suicide, euthanasia, and extended life support.

In regard to abortion, the ongoing debates indicate a tendency toward prohibition among Theravada Buddhists and a more accommodating approach among Japanese and Western Buddhists in the US. The very first Buddhist precept is "to abstain from taking life." Hence based on this precept, the practice of abortion is prohibited. Taking the life of the fetus by mothers or physicians, therefore, may result in bad karma. However, the clinical situation is often complex and may require further nuance of this prohibition. In Buddhism, being is nothing but a combination of consciousness and the physical component. When the body lacks consciousness, being does not exist (Barnhart 1997). Therefore, there is no "being" at conception. Being only emerges during a later development. However, there are those who believe that being exists at conception. Regardless, the emergence of the concept of being is not the only consideration in this issue of abortion (Keown 2020).

Many Buddhists believe that intention must be taken into consideration. Here, it is not purely the act of killing that determines one's karma. If compassion forms the intention of the act then it becomes the source that dictates one's karma. Hence in a situation where abortion may be needed to save the mother's life, this act of abortion may be viewed as one of compassion (Hughes 2007: 129). Viewing the issue from the perspective of intention helps to realize that careless and unmindful sexual engagement that may result in pregnancy and hence abortion will certainly result in negative karma.

Another important factor to be considered is the hierarchy of self in Buddhism. Based on the understanding of karma, not all beings have the same moral status. Hence a more fully developed consciousness, such as that of the mother, may hold a higher moral status than that which is less developed, such as the fetus (Hughes & Keown 1995). Losing either the mother or the child is considered tragic, but when practitioners are forced to save one over the other, this Buddhist concept of hierarchy can assist in dealing with difficult decisions. As healthcare providers, it is important to understand Buddhists' approach to abortion while being conscious of the various possible interpretations. Understanding patients and making appropriate inquiry can help determine the best course of action. According to the Dalai Lama:

Of course, abortion, from a Buddhist viewpoint, is an act of killing and is negative, generally speaking. But it depends on the circumstances. If the unborn child will be retarded or if the birth will create serious problems for the parent, these are cases where there can be an exception. I think abortion should be approved or disapproved according to each circumstance.

(Dreifus 1993: 2)

Death and dying

In Buddhism, the dying process is one of the most essential because what happens at this stage plays a significant role in determining life after death. Healthcare professionals can be instrumental in assisting Buddhist patients through this important transition by accommodating their felt needs in the final stage of life. This may be achieved through practicing meditation, reciting Buddhist texts, contemplating the teachings of the Buddha, coming to terms with death, and generating positive thoughts. These practices are possible for patients when the mind is in a state of consciousness. The question is: when does consciousness cease? Some debate exists surrounding the question of when the self ceases to exist because a person, in Buddhist thought, exists only where there is a combination between consciousness and the body (Becker 1990).

There are a number of perspectives on this issue. According to Venerable Mettanando Bhikkhu (1991: 206–207), death occurs in two stages, namely, the lack of high functioning consciousness and the cessation of physical function. When there is an irreversible loss of high-level consciousness (when a patient becomes permanently unconscious), it is believed that this consciousness has withdrawn into the interior aspect of the individual. But the death designation is given only when physical death takes place as indicated by the lack of activity of the entire brain, both upper and lower level:

> Significantly, if the patient is on life-support, such as a respirator, which is doing the job of the lungs although there is no further stimulus to the lungs from the brain-stem, the patient can be considered clinically dead. All the reflexes – pupil dilation, swallowing, and breathing – need to be tested and found negative before the patient can be declared physically dead.

(Mettanando 1991: 206)

Mettanando Bhikkhu makes a distinction between active life termination and withholding treatment. "In a patient for whom the brainstem is no longer driving the bodily functions, life support is no longer needed" because it is in accord with the definition of clinical death (Mettanando 1991: 210). Hence withholding life support is permissible when a person meets the criteria of clinical death.

In Buddhism, there is generally no unifying agreement in relation to euthanasia except that most Buddhists do not practice involuntary euthanasia (termination of life against the will of the patient). There are, however, differing opinions relating to voluntary (when a person makes the decision to end his/her life) and non-voluntary euthanasia (when a person is not capable of making the decision). For most Buddhists, voluntary euthanasia may be perceived as causing bad karma and thus is viewed unfavorably. While there were cases of Buddhist monks voluntarily ending their lives, they took place under exceptional circumstances. Regarding non-voluntary euthanasia, Mettanando believes that termination of life support is possible when all the reflexes such as pupil dilation, swallowing, and breathing are no longer functioning.

Table 6.1 Dos and don'ts

Dos	Don'ts
1. Pay attention to religious items or sacred threads on patients.	1. Do not remove religious items from patients without permission.
2. Be aware of the role of karma in understanding health and sickness.	2. Do not touch Buddhist monks (for female caregivers) except when they need medical care. Even then, female caregivers should request permission before any form of physical contact.
3. Be aware that clarity of thought prior to death is important since it plays a significant role in determining life after this present death.	3. Do not offer beef to Mahayana Buddhists who worship Guan Yin (goddess of mercy).
4. Permit the use of religious ceremonies/ rituals.	4. Do not invite monks from a tradition different from that of the patient's to perform a religious ceremony.
5. Be aware that Buddhist caregivers are reluctant to perform any treatment that they themselves might consider to result in bad karma.	

When dealing with a deceased patient, Buddhists often let the body rest for two hours before taking any step to transfer the body. Traditionally, a Buddhist monk with incense will lead the body of the deceased to the transportation vehicle and remain with the body until arrival at the temple. The length of the funeral service can last up to one week depending on the status and the finances of family members. It is believed that the soul of the deceased will remain near the body for up to three days. The chanting during the service aims at reminding friends and relatives that death is a part of life; it is something we all have to accept. The service ends with cremation, a reminder that all our basic elements (earth, water, wind, and fire) will return to their original forms.

Conclusion

Buddhism teaches that our ignorance regarding the true nature of human beings leads to suffering. The goal of Buddhism is to help people realize the nature of reality and thus be liberated from suffering through acquiring right understanding and through practicing moderation, compassion, meditation, and other beneficial ways of living in accord with the teachings of the Buddha. In matters relating to health, Buddhism emphasizes harmonious balance of the mind, body, emotions, and spirituality. This balance is made possible when one rightly understands the cause of suffering and the ways that can lead to liberation from the cycle of suffering. Because of the importance of the mind–body connection in Buddhism, caregiver awareness of patient spirituality and practice coupled with a nuanced understanding of karma can help facilitate both physical and spiritual recovery for Buddhists.

Case study #1

Ruthanne was 45 years old when she came to the emergency department with a persistent, acute cough. She was admitted to the hospital ICU with a diagnosis of advanced lung cancer. She soon required mechanical ventilation and consulted with a palliative care specialist who recommended comfort-focused care given her advanced stage of cancer.

The patient left her religious affiliation blank on her intake form. To best meet the patient's needs, the Medical Resident caring for Ruthanne, herself a Buddhist, asked the patient and her mother about the patient's religious affiliation. Offended by the question, the patient's mother responded, "It's none of your business."

After Ruthanne had been hospitalized for a week, she and her mother informed the Resident that she wanted to discontinue ventilatory support. Her lungs were unable to support her without mechanical ventilation. The hospital referred to this as "compassionate extubation," knowing that death would come within minutes to hours after extubation. The Resident made sure Ruthanne and her mother knew what it meant to stop the ventilator.

The Resident caring for Ruthanne was distressed by the request. Ruthanne was her first patient to request compassionate extubation and as a Buddhist she realized she may have some innate biases against discontinuing artificial life-sustaining therapies like a vent. Feeling a bit unsure, the Resident sought the counsel of her Chief Medical Resident, wondering if she could or should be excused from implementing Ruthanne's decision.

Questions for reflection

1. What convictions and beliefs related to the Resident's Buddhist faith could be the foundation of her spiritual distress? Where would you suggest she seek support?
2. Is it important for medical providers to inquire about the spiritual/religious backgrounds of their patients nearing the end of life?
3. Can a physician recuse her/himself from the care of a patient?
4. Does the removal of a ventilator at the patient's request constitute physician assisted suicide?

*Submitted by Garrett Potts

Case study #2

A 30-year-old female presented to the emergency department with intense leg pain after she slipped down a flight of stairs. The patient had no prior health history, lived alone, and identified as Buddhist on her intake form. Upon admission, the patient tearfully expressed to the nurse that, on a scale of 1–10, her level of pain was a 10. The nurse conveyed this to the physician who, after initial examination, suspected that she had a fractured femur. The doctor placed orders for pain medication as well as X-rays.

When the patient heard this plan, she responded: "I will not take any Western drugs." The doctor asked the patient what she meant by her comment, and she clarified that her religion "did not permit any form of intoxication," even if Westerners call it "medicine."

Questions for reflection

1. How might the provider solicit more information about the patient's reservations regarding medication and its potential psychoactive side effects?
2. What spiritual and non-pharmacological practices do some Buddhists utilize to navigate pain?
3. How could the provider and interdisciplinary team address the patient's pain?

4. Two weeks later, this provider cares for another Buddhist patient who is very willing to take pain medication for a similar injury. Knowing you have taken a course in World Religions, the physician asks you to help her understand. What would you say?

*Submitted by Joset Brown

Glossary

Anatta Used to denote a sense of no-self; that is, there is no real self. What we term "self" is an illusion.

Annica Referring to impermanence, this term notes that everything in this life is in the state of impermanence.

Avijja Refers to our ignorance which ultimately leads us to the cycle of incarnation.

Dukkha Refers to the sense of suffering that is central to the religion of Buddhism; the Buddha taught that to exist is to suffer.

Paticcasamuppada The law of dependent origination seeking to explain the cycle of life.

Tanha Close to the concept of desire. Desire always leads to attachment, and attachment to being.

Note

1 Supaporn Naewbood, one of the original authors of this chapter, was unable to be involved in the update for this third edition.

Bibliography

Barnhart, M. (1997) "Buddhism and the Morality of Abortion," *Journal of Buddhist Ethics*, 5. http://blogs.dickinson.edu/buddhistethics/2010/04/08/buddhism-and-the-morality-of-abortion/

Becker, CB. (1990) "Buddhist Views of Suicide and Euthanasia," *Philosophy East and West*, 40: 543–556.

Buddha Dharma Association and BuddhaNet (n.d.). "Statistics on the Major Branches of Buddhism." www.buddhanet.net/e-learning/history/bstats_b.htm

Dhammacakkappavattana Sutta (1993) "Setting the Wheel of Dhamma in Motion" (Thanissaro Bhikkhu, Trans.). www.accesstoinsight.org/tipitaka/sn/sn56/sn56.011.than.html

Dammapada (n.d.). *Oceanlibrary*. https://oceanlibrary.com/dhammapada_buddha/

Dreifus, C. (1993) "The Dalai Lama," New York Times, November 28, 1993, p. 2.

Hewapathirane, D. (2004) "Buddhism, Health and Wellbeing," *Wisdom*, 9(1): 6–8.

Hughes, J. (2007) "Buddhist Bioethics," in Ashcroft, RE., Dawson, A., Draper, H., and McMillan, JR. (eds) *Principles of Health Care Ethics* (pp. 127–134). New York: John Wiley & Sons.

Hughes, J., and Keown, D. (1995) "Buddhism and Medical Ethics: A Bibliographic Introduction," *Journal of Buddhist Ethics*, 2. www.researchgate.net/publication/239843678_Buddhism_and_Medical_Ethics_A_Bibliographic_Introduction

Kantharadussadee-Triamchaisri, S., Tengtrisron, C., Mahaweerawatana, U., Powatana, A., Permpornsakul, C., and Smitrakasetrin, S. (2004) *Mind-Spiritual Exercise and Healing among HIV/AIDS Patients in Thailand*. Bangkok: Ministry of Health.

Keown, D. (2020) "Abortion," *Buddhist Ethics: A Very Short Introduction*, 2nd ed., online edn. Oxford: Oxford Academic. https://doi.org/10.1093/actrade/9780198850052.003.0006

Mark, JJ. (2020) "A Short History of the Buddhist Schools," *World History Encyclopedia*. www.worldhistory.org/article/492/a-short-history-of-the-buddhist-schools/

Matthews, W. (1999) *World Religions*, 3rd ed. Belmont, CA: Wadsworth.

Mettanando, B. (1991) "Buddhist Ethics in the Practice of Medicine," in Fu, CW. and Wawrytho, SA. (eds) *Buddhist Ethics and Modern Society: An International Symposium* (pp. 195–213). New York: Greenwood.

Ratanakul, P. (2004) "Buddhism, Health and Disease," *Eubios: Journal of Asian and International Bioethics*, 15: 162–164.

Reynolds, FE., Kitagawa, JM., Nakamura, H., and Tucci, G., Snellgrove, DL., and Lopez, DS. (2023) "Buddhism," *Encyclopedia Britannica*. www.britannica.com/topic/Buddhism

Samyuta Nikaya (2000) (Bhikku Bodhi, Trans). https://obo.genaud.net/dhamma-vinaya/wp/sn/03_kv/sn03.22.026.bodh.wp.htm

Wiist, WH., Sullivan, BM., St. George, DM., and Wayment, HA. (2012) "Buddhists' Religious and Health Practices," *Journal of Religion and Health*, 51(1): 132–147. www.jstor.org/stable/41349872

Wijesinghe, S. (2013) *Role of Buddhist Spiritual Practice in the Lives and health of Buddhist Nuns Living with a Chronic Illness in Sri Lanka* [Doctoral dissertation, University of NewMexico]. UNM Repository. https://digitalrepository.unm.edu/nurs_etds/15

World Population Review (2022) *Buddhist Countries*. https://worldpopulationreview.com/country-rankings/buddhist-countries

7 Jainism

Whitny Braun de Lobatón

All breathing, existing, living, sentient creatures should not be slain, nor treated with violence, nor abused, nor tormented, nor driven away.

(*Mahāvirā*, from *Ācharanga Sutra* 1996: 262)

Introduction

For Jains time is eternal and cyclical. There is no beginning and there will be no end. The bodies of all life forms are but physical vessels for the eternal soul or the *jivā*. Each soul will move from physical body to physical body again and again throughout time until the soul can limit the amount of *karma* accrued. This allows their soul to break free from the prison of the physical body and float to the top of the universe where it can reside for all time in a formless, blissful, omnipotent state, free from the cycle of reincarnation forever.

In Jainism there is but one maxim, that each soul must strive to live by: Ahimsa or non-violence. Jains strive to pass through this life leaving as little a mark as possible. For Jains at the end of their lives they want to leave the world with the slightest "violence footprint" possible.

Demographics

Jains can be found operating in the most elite circles of business, banking, politics, academia, and science. And then you will find them living, by choice, in abject poverty and austerity seeking to free themselves of all the trappings of modern life. Jains who exist somewhere in the middle of the economic spectrum are rare.

Accurate census data regarding Jain communities can be difficult to obtain as Jains are often simply calculated into more general categories such as "Hindu" or "Other," but there should be no mistaking the fact that Jainism is a distinct philosophical tradition. In 2011 it was estimated that there were just under five million Jains in the world with approximately 4.2 million living in the religion's country of origin, India. Unfortunately, the COVID-19 pandemic has delayed further census work that would yield current numbers (Census of India 2011). While the bulk of the Jain population can be found in South Asia there are sizable diaspora communities across the globe. Africa is home to approximately 20,000 Jains with major concentrations in Kenya and South Africa (Dundas 2002: 271). Approximately 65,000 Jains reside in the United Kingdom and

DOI: 10.4324/9781003288862-7

an estimated 150,000 practicing Jains reside in the United States (Thomas 2019; Lee 2010: 487–488). One of the most prominent diaspora communities (approximately 15,000) are the Jains of Antwerp, Belgium who are deeply involved in the precious stone trade. Economists estimate that this population now controls up to two-thirds of the wholesale diamond trade in this international commercial hub (Kapur 2010: 104).

History

The Jain philosophy and religion is believed by its followers to be eternal. There is no creation myth nor is there an apocalyptic future foretold. Instead, Jains believe that civilizations ebb and flow and there have been times in the past and will be times in the future when the truth of Jainism will be known and then disappear into the mists of history again. But the purity and the truth of Jainism will never perish or go extinct. And from time to time throughout the ages 24 *Tīrthaṅkaras*, translated as "ford makers" or prophets, appear to share the eternal wisdom of Jain philosophy with humanity. They appear in definite and fixed intervals as perfect beings that serve as great teachers and exemplars (Glasenapp 1999: 15).

In known human history, which Jains understand as just one of an endless series of epochs, 24 *Tīrthaṅkaras* have been recorded. The first of these is the mythical figure of Lord Ṛṣabha also known as Ādinātha (Baya 2007: 256), who may have been a historical figure of the Indus Valley Civilization dating as far back as 3,300 BCE. The earliest of the *Tīrthaṅkaras* that can be reliably dated as a historical figure is the 23rd, Pārśvanātha, who is believed to have lived circa 877–777 BCE. Whether or not Ādinātha or Pārśvanātha can be credited as being the founders of Jainism in the modern world is debatable. From the Jain perspective there can be no founder of Jainism as it is an eternal truth and not the teachings of one man. From the perspective of the historical academy the title of founder of the faith traditionally belongs to a man who lived from 599 BCE–527 BCE known as Mahāvīra.

There is little doubt that Mahāvīra was a historical figure. Not only is his existence documented in many Jain writings, but he is also referenced in Buddhist scriptures as a contemporary of Gautama Buddha (Glasenapp 1999: 16). He was born Vardhamāna, the son of a *Kṣatriya* named Siddhārtha and his wife Triśalā in the Kuṇḍagrāma, located in the present-day Indian state of Bihar. His father, as *Rājā*, provided him with a life of privilege and opulence, a marriage to a princess who bore him a daughter, and all the luxuries he desired.

By his 30th year of life, he renounced his royal privilege and set off on his own (Jaini 1998: 11). He first traveled to an area of wilderness called Ṣandavana and fasted for two and a half days under an Aśoka tree. According to the *Śvetambara* tradition he donned robes of *deva-dūṣya* or divine cloth and proceeded to pull out his hair in five tufts in the ritual known as *kesá-loca* (Jaini 1998: 12). He then shed his robes so as to purge himself of any possessions and became a nude itinerant monk wandering the countryside.

He first joined the order of ascetics believed by historians to have been founded on the teachings of Pārśvanātha near his hometown but found that they did not live in austere enough conditions and chose to wander on his own. For 12 years he walked the area of the Ganges River Basin and was the subject of scorn, ridicule, and mockery for his nudity and ascetic practices. But, by the end of his 12th year of itinerant preaching, he attained omniscience (*kevala jñana*) while sitting under a tree on the banks of the Rjupālikā River. It was in this moment of conquering his passions and mental frailties that he earned the title of Mahāvīra or "the great hero" as he assumed the role of an *arihant*, a venerable person who would become the 24th *Tīrthaṅkara*.

Upon accession to the role of *Tīrthaṅkara* he made it his duty to revive the teachings of Pārśvanātha. He set out on foot through the countryside of Bihar and for the next 30 years preached to both men and women of all walks of life. It is believed that he died in 527 BCE at the age of 72 after having taken the vow of *Sallekhanā* and achieved *mokṣa;* complete liberation, thus ascending to the apex of the universe to exist for all eternity in the abode of the *Siddhas* (*Siddhaloka*) in a perfect, formless, genderless state.

According to tradition Mahāvīra had converted 14,000 monks, 36,000 nuns, 159,000 lay men, and 318,000 lay women to the Jain system of belief by the time of his death (Glasenapp 1999: 39). It is commonly believed that Mahāvīra passed away within the lifetime of the Buddha and in the years following both of their deaths, Jainism and Buddhism emerged as the premiere *Śramanic* faiths of the Vedic period in northern India.

The Jain community split into two main sectarian groups: *Digambaras* and *Śvetāmbaras*. The *Digambaras* are the "sky clad" sect known for their male ascetics who give up clothing and live as itinerant monks in the nude. The *Digambaras* are further divided into at least three distinct sectarian groups: the *Digambara Terapatha* of *Śuddhāmnāya*, the *Bispanth*, and the *Samaiyā* (Jain 1999: 5). The *Śvetāmbaras* are the "white clad" sect known for their ascetics wearing simple white robes and often a cloth across their mouths called a *muphatti* to prevent the accidental inhalation of microscopic life. The *Śvetāmbaras* are further divided into sub-sects: the *Murtipujaka (Deravasi)*, the *Sthānakavāsi*, and the *Terapanthi*. There are several differences in the beliefs and practices of the two sects (*Digambaras* and *Śvetāmbaras*) but perhaps the most notable, besides the differences in their appearance and attitudes toward idol worship and the historical timeline, is that *Digambaras* hold that all 24 of the *Tīrthaṅkaras* were men. Additionally, they believe that only men can achieve *mokṣa* whereas the *Śvetāmbaras* believe that women can achieve *mokṣa*, entering the *siddha* state directly from the form of a human woman. The *Śvetāmbaras* believe that the 19th *Tīrthankara* was a woman named Māllīnātha (Jaini 1998: 40). It is possible that because of this *Śvetāmbaras* belief that women can achieve *mokṣa*, more *Śvetāmbara* women are recorded as engaging in *Sallekhanā*.

There is debate as to how the schism between the two main sects in Jainism came about. One theory is that the once homogenous population split about two centuries after the death of Mahāvīra around the year 290 BCE when the ācāryaSri Bhadrabāhu migrated, along with 12,000 ascetics and lay followers from Pāṭaliputra to the state of Karnataka in the South of India in a desperate attempt to avoid a famine. It is said that Bhadrabāhu passed away before a return to Bihar was possible and when a few followers did return they found that many of the practices of their original community had changed under the leadership of Sthūlabhadra, including the wearing of clothing. Unable to accept these changes, the group that had left Pāṭaliputra under Bhadrabāhu became the *Digambaras* and those who followed the leadership of Sthūlabhadra became the *Śvetambaras* (Jaini 1998: 5). This division was cemented at the Council of Vallabhi in the fifth century CE (Kelting 2003: 640).

Beliefs and practices

One aspect of Jain doctrine that distinguishes it from most other religions is that in the last three millennia it has experienced very little dogmatic development when compared to the Abrahamic or even other Dharmic traditions (Glasenapp 1999: 164). After Mahāvīra's death, his disciples, the *Gaṇadharas*, recorded his teachings and a lineage of Jain scholars was established that produced the works that continue to form the corpus of the Jain canons. Thus, the practices prescribed for the aspirant who wishes to achieve a good death have remained almost unchanged through the centuries.

Jain soteriology can only be understood in the context of Jain cosmology. Jainism does not espouse that the universe (*loka*) was created by an intelligent, divine being but rather describes the universe as an eternal, physical constant, made up of six *dravya* or substances that also have always been and always will be. These *dravya* are sentient beings or souls (*jīva*), non-sentient matter (*pudgala*), energy of motion (*dharma*), the principle of rest (*adharma*), space (*ākāśa*), and time (*kāla*).

The cosmos is a giant space where the abode of the liberated souls, the heavens where the gods reside, the middle world, which contains the realm of men, and the seven levels of hell exist. This universe is conceptualized in the shape of a man with arms bent, resting on the hips and feet planted apart. Outside of this *loka* there is nothing but a giant void filled with strong winds (Dundas 2002: 90).

Again, this *loka* is not the work of a conscious, divine entity. It has no beginning and no end and is an eternal physical cosmos, thus there is no eschatological view in Jainism. In the *loka* there are three realms that exist below the supreme abode of the *Siddhas*: the infernal, terrestrial, and celestial. Only those *jīva* who are born into the realm of men can theoretically hope to strive for deliverance from their earthly physical form.

The infernal realm or *Naraka* exists at the bottom of the *loka* where there are seven levels of hell. As one goes deeper through the levels of hell the geographical expanse of each gets broader, and the beings that exist in these realms are characterized by a dark soul coloring (*parināma*) and commit violence against each other causing pain and suffering. Below the bottommost hell there are no forms of life (Shah 2000: 127). The beings that exist in these hells are not born in the same way that humans are born in the middle earth. They are oddly born by spontaneously manifesting from holes in the walls and falling into the hell. These beings are hermaphrodites and fully conscious of their suffering (Shah 2000: 260).

Located above the hellish realms is the circular middle realm known as middle *loka* or *Madhyaloka* and in the center of this terrestrial realm there are numerous oceans and countless continents rising from the waters. The continents derive their names because of their unique characteristics. The oceans are named for the liquids that their water resembles (Shah 2000: 253). Rising from the center of this middle earth is Mount Meru. The middle world has a central continent of *Jambūdvīpa*, translated as "The Island of the Roseapple Tree," forming with the adjacent continent of *Dhātakīkhaṇḍa* and half of the continent nearest to it, *Puskaradvīpa*, to create the abode of humankind (Dundas 2002: 91). *Jambūdvīpa* is surrounded by an imposing wall built entirely of diamonds and a large lotus-terrace with ponds built from precious stones. There is also said to be a large gate wrought from gold and jewels with four entry points protected by deities (Glasenapp 1999: 254). Outside these gates is the abode of humankind.

Those who conquer *saṁsāra* (the cycle of birth, death, and rebirth) and travel to the abode of the *Siddhas* do so from the abode of humankind. However, there is another realm above the middle realm where the celestial beings reside.

Above the middle world is a series of heavens, which increase in size and brightness and beauty, and where gods and goddesses exist. This realm is called the *devloka*. These gods are divided into four *nikāyas* or species: *Bhavanapati*, *Vyantara*, *Jyotiṣka*, and *Vaimānika* (Glasenapp 1999: 147). While the hellish beings are greyish in color the heavenly beings enjoy light bodily colors. Among the *Vaimānikas* the gods have a yellow bodily color and those gods who live in the third up to the fifth heavens have a red form, while all gods residing in the sixth heaven up to the *sarvārthasiddha* (celestial beings that exist in a higher cosmic realm) have white bodies (Glasenapp 1999: 164).

Ultimately gods and goddesses must be reborn in the middle world as men or women to continue on the path to *mokṣa* so their time in the celestial realm is somewhat bittersweet in that they will need to leave that heavenly abode to continue their spiritual journey. Some of these gods and goddesses can experience sexual enjoyment but that enjoyment will ultimately lead to their fall. The greater the intensity of the sexual passion the greater their mental desire, and the greater the desire the harder it is to satisfy it. Thus, a struggle ensues for the god that will ultimately result in the god being reborn in human form. The higher up in the levels of heaven a god resides the larger their physical form, the longer their life and the more pleasure they feel, even though they are less arrogant (Shah 2000: 162–163).

Above the heavens and at the end of the upward climb up the levels of the *loka* is the *Īsatprāgbhāra*, or "slightly curving place" (Dundas 2002: 91) where the liberated souls exist, experiencing pure knowledge, energy, and bliss, having broken through the cycles of *saṁsāra*, freeing themselves from the pain of birth, death, and rebirth.

Health and disease

In Jain philosophy, as long as the soul remains in its mundane unenlightened existence, decay, disease, and death are certain. Life is not thought of as a pleasant experience. The *Uttarādhyayanasūtra*, one of the fundamental textual sources used in the instruction of Jain monastics, says that "birth, death, decay, and disease are sorrows, the mundane existence itself is full of sorrow, where the living beings feel miserable." Further, the *Ādi Śaṅkarācārya*, an eight century Vedic scholar's writing's posit that repeated births and deaths, the process known as *saṁsāra*, and lying in the wombs of mothers is very painful.

The death of humans and animals occurs when the being has reached the quantum of life allotted to it by its *karma*. This death occurs as a result of a specific cause known as an *upakrama* but for Gods and hellish beings death takes place spontaneously and the *jivā* is carried along on its spiritual journey by the force of *anupūrvināmakarma*, the cosmic calculator of sorts that determines karmic destiny and reckons the location of rebirth. This time between death and rebirth is infinitesimally short and known as *vigrahakāla* (Glasenapp 1999: 201).

The ultimate spiritual desire for the Jains has been to find a way to be set free from physical pain and fear that is inherent in the form of a living being. Life is characterized by fear and suffering with the end result of death and to be free of this cycle of violence and pain is the supreme wish. The Jain *Tīrthaṅkaras* developed and shared a unique way to overcome this fear and the accompanying misery of life by teaching a practice which allowed a person to approach death voluntarily in a state of equanimity. They prescribed a ritual in which a person sheds the *karma* that weighs down their soul and achieves *moksha* or liberation of the soul. This concept is unique to the Jain philosophy and is referred to as *Samādhimaraṇa*, the peaceful death and the ritual itself is popularly known as *Sallekhanā* (Glasenapp 1999: 200).

Ultimately each soul needs to purge itself of *karma* in order to achieve spiritual deliverance or *mokṣa*. But there are steps on the journey to *mokṣa*. The individual should strive for right belief, right knowledge, and right conduct. By striving to perfect the soul the individual can work toward achieving enlightenment and becoming a *kevalin*. However, being a *kevalin* and enjoying omniscience does not immediately seal one's fate as having achieved liberation. Upon attaining enlightenment the individual may live for quite some time engaging in mental and physical activities such as walking, preaching, and meditation. However, no new *karma* is accrued at this time and the individual is not committing any acts of violence (Dundas 2002: 104).

Paul Dundas explains the next step in the process of moving from enlightenment to liberation as follows:

> It is necessary for life karma to run its course before final deliverance can be gained. From the time of the scriptural texts, Jain theoreticians claimed that is might be necessary for the enlightened person, or *kevalin*, to perform an expulsion (*samudghāta*) of karmic particles in order to equalize experience karma, which has been generally bound more intensely than any other type, with life karma. This strange process is affected by the kevalin expanding the *jīva* for the short duration of eight instants, to the height and width of the *loka* in a variety of temporarily assumed shapes, whereupon, after ejecting karmic particles in the same way as dust is shaken off an open sheet which is then refolded, it subsequently returns to the confines of the human body. This ensures that the non-harming karmas will quickly reach their end and the *kevalin* then starts to run down the operation of the mind, body and speech until all natural functioning ceases.
>
> (2002: 104)

The *kevalin* then articulates five verses, and the four non-harming *karmas* disappear. The *jivā* becomes free from its body or physical prison and then ascends through the *loka* instantaneously and enters the abode of the *Siddhas* at the top of the universe. Here in the abode of the *Siddhas* the *jivā* will exist in a perfect, peaceful, genderless state experiencing only bliss.

Sallekhanā, *Santhārā*, or *Samādhimaraṇa*, all terms used in the Jain religion to describe a ritualistic, voluntary, and peaceful death, are discussed in the Jain canonical texts. This end of life ritual is regarded as one of the most prestigious rights of passage in the Jain code of conduct. Jain canonical lore is full of prescriptions for and instances of individuals, both monastics and laity, choosing this journey to voluntary death in order to culminate their spiritual journey in this lifetime. It serves as the supreme expression of Jain faith and as a means to reach liberation of the soul.

Death and dying

In the broadest sense of Jain philosophy an eternal soul (*jivā*) is subject to the cycle of birth, death, and rebirth (*saṃsāra*). When in a physical form, particularly a human form, the worth of the body that houses the soul is based on utility. The physical body is a tool or the conduit by which the soul seeks out knowledge and enlightenment and proceeds on its spiritual journey. When the physical body begins to fail and is more of a burden than an asset, the Jain canons teach that the enlightened aspirant is best served by accepting that their body is but a temporary vessel and that death is a natural progression and thus it is preferable to embrace death rather than hang on to life. The Jain canons in essence suggest that rather than allowing the grim specter of death to stalk you, as the aspirant you give up life-sustaining practices such as eating and drinking and meet death with a posture of openness. And in this psychological acceptance of death, you adopt a position or attitude of equanimity toward death.

The *Tattvārthasutra*, compiled in the fifth century BCE, represents the earliest known compendium of Jain doctrinal beliefs. The author of this massive work was the chief disciple of Lord Mahāvīra, a man named Umāsvati, who created a "handbook for understanding the meaning of the basic truths" (Glasenapp 1999: 126) in which he describes 14 stages through which a soul must travel to reach the end point of *mokṣa* or liberation upon death. These 14 phases are known as the *Guasthāna* or "levels of virtue" and are likened to the rungs of a ladder (Jaini 1998: 141). One may climb up or down on the ladder depending on their actions but in order to achieve the ultimate goal of transcending the cycle of *saṁsāra* a *jivā* must at some point move sequentially up the ladder, through the 14 stages.

Each higher stage moves the practitioner from various states of ignorance, passion, bad conduct, and more *karma* to states of omniscience, less passion, perfect conduct, and decreasing amounts of *karma* until there is no *karma* left at all. This path to perfection is sometimes called the "path of purification" (Jaini 1998: 141).

Until omniscience is gained at the top of the ladder upon becoming a *kevalin*, a person cannot claim to know the whole truth of reality, so that every assertion must be qualified as a partial truth. True understanding of the nature of existence remains elusive to all until omniscience is achieved.

The linguistic origin of the word *Sallekhanā* in Prakrit has the commonly accepted definition of "properly thinning out the passions of the body" (Jaini 1998: 229). It is the combination of the prefix *sam* meaning "proper" and *lekhanā* that translates as "reducing the physical body." Any Jain who is faced with ailments can approach their guru and express their wish to take the vow of *Sallekhanā*. They do so by saying the words:

> Please instruct me sir. I have come forward to seek…*Sallekhanā*, (the vow of) which will remain in force as long as I live. I am free of all doubts and anxieties in this matter. I renounce, from now until the moment of my last breath, food and drink of all kinds.
> (Jaini 1998: 229)

Assuming that permission is granted, the person either decides independently or consults with their physician as to the approximate amount of time he or she has left to live and then develops a program of fasting to coincide with their vow of *Sallekhanā*. While the philosophical rationale surrounding *Sallekhanā* has remained virtually unchanged through the centuries, one adaption that is evolving is that more Jains are consulting their physician for an opinion and assistance in formulating a timetable for *Sallekhanā*. At any time and at any stage along the human wellness spectrum an individual may begin the ritual. Ideally, the *Sallekhanā* undertaken by the perfectly healthy person of sound mind and body is the most spiritually rewarding form, and is known as *Prāyopagamana* (Settar 2017: 12–13).

A member of the laity who accepts the vow gives up all personal relationships and possessions. He or she forgives all and asks for the pardon of all their sins (Sogani 2005: 231). During this period all negative emotion should be eliminated. It must also be understood that if they are committing to *Sallekhanā* in response to a terminal diagnosis, and if their disease were to be cured, or their diagnosis found to be incorrect, the vow of *Sallekhanā* may not be rescinded.

Sallekhanā is typically done in the family home or in a fasting hall known as a *dharmaśala*. Historically though, such as in the case of Lord Mahāvīra, it was undertaken in a remote space in nature. While a person practices *Sallekhanā* they have no worldly responsibilities. They turn all property over to their family and sequester themselves to avoid distraction. Relatives often publicize the event by taking out ads in local newspapers. When the person eventually dies it is not uncommon for the body to be ornately decorated and paraded through the community before cremation.

The practice of ending one's life through fasting in the pursuit of non-violence is not unique to the Jains (Keown 1999: 393). What is distinctive is that it is so entrenched in the culture and is practiced on such a consistent basis (Laidlaw 2005: 181). Not every Jain takes the vow of *Sallekhanā*, but all Jains have the option available to them. What makes *Sallekhanā* more remarkable is that while this death ritual is prescribed as a necessary step on the path to liberation all Jains know that if they take the vow, it will not result in liberation for them at this time. At best they hope that making the choice to take the vow of *Sallekhanā* results in reincarnation in a better form and place in the next life.

Samādhimaraṇa, Sallekhanā, and Santhārā

While the terms *Samādhimaraṇa* and *Sallekhanā* are frequently used interchangeably, they have distinctly different grammatical and conceptual nuances. *Samādhimaraṇa* is a state of being, a peaceful death and a dispassionate end. It is the experience of death itself, a singular point in time. *Sallekhanā* is a vow followed by a process; a ritual journey one embarks on to achieve *Samādhimaraṇa* (Baya 2007: 43).

The peaceful death and the journey toward achieving it were perhaps developed as a response to the truth written in the *Daśavaikālika Sutra* which says ever so simply, "Everyone wants to live and none wants to die" (*Daśavaikālika* 6.10, Bhadrabahu 1973: 98). This may be true enough but as death is inevitable the great Jain thinkers had to philosophize a response to this existential woe. Thus, they sought to create and apply a moral value and ethical framework to the process of death and dying and developed a code that prescribes conquering the fear of death in a fully engaged manner.

This process of accepting death, of psychologically preparing oneself to voluntarily end one's life, should ideally result in the person looking back on a life of piety and therefore having no fear because they are assured of a good reincarnation. The *Tattvārthasūtra* says that the aspirant should think, "I have followed the path of virtue and thus I do not fear death" (*Tattvārthasūtra* 7.22, Jain 2018: 417). Conversely one who has lived a sinful life full of worldly attachments dies fretfully, fearing death for fear of being reborn in hellish circumstances or as an animal (*Ātur Pratyākhyān* 63, Suriji 2002: 68).

The Jain emphasis on the primary importance of conduct in achieving spiritual liberation has led to the development of a highly rigorous code of monastic practices and a very stringent code of conduct for its laity. Severe penance as a means of purging accumulated *karma* from the soul is prescribed for all followers of the Jain religion. The volumes of the *Ardhamāgadhī* canonical works are filled with the concept and detailed procedural descriptions for the attainment of *Samādhimaraṇa* by *Sallekhanā*.

There are linguistic nuances to the terms *Sallekhanā* and *Santhārā* and there are distinctions in how they should be used and the spiritual implications they connote.

Sallekhanā

In the *Sthānāṅga Vṛtti*, the Ācārya Abhayadevasūri said that *Sallekhanā* is, "The activity by which the body is weakened, and passions are overcome" (*Maranassabihemi* 63, Baya 2007: 351). The *Jñātā-dharmakathā-sūtra Vṛtti* echoes the same definition (*Jñātādharmakathāṅga* 1/1 Vṛtti 1981: 658). Other works give a slightly different linguistic allusion describing *Sallekhanā* as the "peeling off of the passions" of the body and the forfeiting bodily strength in order to strengthen the spirit. To weaken the physical body is *Dravya Sallekhanā* while to overcome the passions of the body is *Bhāva Sallekhanā*. Since Jain thought considers the body a prison for the soul and the passions like the chains that hold the soul in its prison it is of paramount importance in Jain belief to weaken these two entities in order to liberate the soul.

Sallekhanā is a continuing practice aimed at weakening the body externally and the passions internally. Thus, *Sallekhanā* can actually be an open-ended form of preparatory penance that trains the aspirant to embrace the final act of death but does not necessarily have to end in death. The penance in and of itself is a spiritually rewarding ritual. The positive death that results from *Sallekhanā* is then called *Samādhimaraṇa*. This sets it apart linguistically and conceptually from *Santhārā*, which is just death. Also, the option of specific periods of time in which to take *Sallekhanā*, such as 12 years, 12 months, or 12 weeks proves that it is an open-ended penance that is not always meant to end in death.

The *Ācārāṅga* is categorical in stating that a monk must gradually reduce his food intake and weaken his body in order to prepare for the end-practice of *Santhārā* when and only when he feels that his body has become incapacitated due to various reasons, and he is unable to bear it any longer. According to the *Ācārya Samantabhadra*, *Antima Māraṇāntika Sallekhanā* must be practiced in cases of acute affliction like famine, extreme old age, and incurable disease (Baya 2007: 49).

Santhārā

Santhārā, unlike the open-ended ritual that *Sallekhanā* can be, is the end practice of embracing voluntary death and end the life. The three types of rigor (*Bhaktapratyākhyāna*, *Inginī*, and *Padapoapagamana*) associated with the final moments of life are associated with the category of *Santhārā*.

Santhārā is considered to be the aspirations of the devout Jain come to fruition after lifelong penance (*Mṛtyu Mahotsava* 2, 2010: 22). But it should be noted that this rigorous lifelong penance is only useful if the aspirant has attained equanimity of mind at the time of death (*Mṛtyu Mahotsava* 23, 2010: 24).

Sallekhanā may be a relatively obscure practice, used by very small subsets of the population, but because of its dramatically different approach to the ending of a person's life it is a potentially problematic ritual for the allopathic medical community to rationalize.

Allopathic medicine has evolved to place sustaining life as the major ethical and moral objective of its practitioners.

While *Sallekhanā* is a ritual native to India its practice is spreading to the United States. Though official numbers are unknown, conversations with members of the Jain community reveal that the occurrence of it is increasing as more Jains immigrate to the United States. In order for the United States to maintain cultural pluralism the medical community needs to become familiar with the rules, rationale, and rituals associated with this practice in order to offer Jain patients in the clinical setting effective holistic care and possibly prevent the abuse of the practice of *Sallekhanā*.

The perception of *Sallekhanā* to an outsider may be macabre. The idea of a person abstaining from food and water may seem torturous and abusive. It would be natural for someone such as a physician, unfamiliar with the practice, to immediately conclude that the person enduring the fast is experiencing discomfort. Then, based on the default position that a healthcare provider offers comfort to a person who is ailing, the physician may try to offer comfort in the form of nutrition or hydration, and when the person declines that offer the physician may interpret the person's choice to fast to death as being symptomatic of mental incapacity. In which case a conflict may arise between the physician, the patient, and the state as to whether that person is practicing religious freedom or demonstrating decisional incapacity that requires they be protected from themselves.

Non-Jain clinicians both in India and the United States can lay the groundwork for an inter-faith and inter-cultural dialogue that could facilitate a reconciliation of the American healthcare system's largely Christian-inspired bioethics with the Jain concept of right knowledge and practice. Would it not break the principle of "do no harm" to deprive a person who believes that their soul will be wounded and their future lives negatively impacted by being prevented from engaging in their religiously sanctioned, ideal form of death?

Conclusion

The normative ethics of *Sallekhanā* constitute a larger and more complicated issue. For healthcare professionals *Sallekhanā* is an ethically and morally troubling practice. If *Sallekhanā* is ever used as a means of coercing the elderly, infirm, or simply unwanted members of the society into suicide, the practice is unquestionably wrong. However, if *Sallekhanā* is a religious ritual and an exercise in personal and patient autonomy that brings comfort to the dying in their final days, then *Sallekhanā* may also be an ethically defensible path toward death.

To outlaw *Sallekhanā* would be unethical as a violation of the right to religious freedom guaranteed not only in the constitutions of the United States and India but by Article 18 of the Universal Declaration of Human Rights. However, in the interest of protecting vulnerable members of the community, both the Jain and global communities' attention must be drawn to *Sallekhanā* to prevent its abuse. For the sake of delivering culturally appropriate counsel and treatment to those members of the Jain community seeking healthcare it is imperative that medical professionals familiarize themselves with the rules, rituals, and rationale of *Sallekhanā*.

Ultimately the argument must be put forth that within Jain communities – whether in India or in the United States or in any liberal democracy – the moral presumption

Table 7.1 Dos and Don'ts

Dos	Don'ts
1. Do encourage a Jain to be open about their faith	1. Don't encourage a Jain to eat meat or take antibiotics
2. Do encourage Jains to ask for a quiet space to practice meditation	2. Don't encourage a Jain to take heroic measures to extend their lifespan
3. Do encourage a Jain to ask for assistance from a palliative care specialist	3. Don't attempt to encourage a Jain to eat if they are fasting
4. Do acknowledge that Jains do not view *Sallekhanā* as suicide	4. Don't encourage a Jain to practice abortion or engage in any other act that could be construed as violence
5. Do acknowledge that some Jains may choose to pursue more aggressive treatment and forego *Sallekhanā*	5. Don't assume that all Jains will choose *Sallekhanā*

should be that *Sallekhanā* is a valid religious ritual of dying and therefore should be legally protected. However, the legal sanctioning of *Sallekhanā* should only occur when chosen by a rational person. Given that *Sallekhanā* is sometimes abused, the person contemplating *Sallekhanā* should be advised of the availability of medical treatment for the condition precipitating consideration of *Sallekhanā*, if such treatment exists, and of the right to forego *Sallekhanā* if the person is experiencing pressure or coercion in any form.

Case study #1

The best chance of survival for a 36-year-old woman with stage 3 ovarian cancer was a hysterectomy followed by radiation and chemotherapy. After discussing her prognosis and treatment options with her family, she told her physicians that she would forgo treatment and instead take the vow of *Sallekhanā* although her husband wanted her to undergo the prescribed treatment.

As a Jain she felt her body was just a physical vessel for her eternal soul. The hysterectomy would require taking antibiotics following the surgery. Because Jains believe that all life forms have eternal souls of equal value, she believed taking antibiotics was a form of genocide, killing the millions of bacteria that live in her body. The chemotherapy and radiation would kill other microbial life forms in her body. Additionally, as a believing Jain, she would not take medicines that contained animal by-products. For instance, a successful surgery would be followed by hormone replacements derived from animal cellular sources.

Resolute in her vow of *Sallekhanā*, she began to experience such debilitating pain from the cancer that her husband arranged for hospice care in their home. In the last month of her life photos of her two children were moved a few feet further away from her bedside each day until they were completely out of sight. She then asked her husband to stop visiting her in her room and allow her to pass away without feeling any emotional attachment. Nine months after receiving her diagnosis, the woman died from renal failure induced by her refusal to eat or drink.

Questions for reflection

1. Is it the place of a physician to question a patient of faith's motives in choosing to forgo treatment for terminal cancer?
2. Does a young mother have an obligation to honor the wishes of her husband and pursue treatment for the sake of the well-being of her children in spite of her spiritual beliefs?
3. Consider the parallel between this patient's belief regarding bacteria and the belief that a fertilized human ovum is entitled to legal protection as a human being. Is the intrinsic value of an organism affected by its size?

*Submitted by Whitny Braun de Lobatón

Case study #2

A Jain couple in their late 30s sought the assistance of a reproductive endocrinologist in the hope of having a child. After less intensive methods failed to work, they proceeded with in vitro fertilization (IVF). Given the details of their case, the physician explained that they would likely produce many viable embryos which increased their chances of a successful pregnancy. However, given the couple's age and past difficulties conceiving, the physician advised that they screen the embryos to rate their genetic quality. They would proceed only with the healthiest embryos leaving the couple with the decision of what to do with the remaining embryos.

The couple was uncomfortable with this path for several reasons:

1. They felt that their embryos would each have a *jivā* or soul.
2. As they only desired one child they knew they would have four choices of what to do with their remaining embryos, a) destroy them, killing the *jivās*, b) keep them perpetually frozen which would effectively thwart the effects of *karma* and progress spiritually, c) donate them for scientific research where they would ultimately be destroyed anyway, or d) give them up for adoption to be gestated by another woman and raised by another family.
3. The IVF process requires using medications and the egg retrieval surgery would require the wife to take antibiotics to prevent possible infection.

Ultimately, they told their endocrinologist that they could not in good conscience go forward with IVF. They had consulted with their religious community and decided against the violence wrought upon their surplus embryos. They could not imagine having their embryos born into other families nor could they navigate their emotional attachment to the surplus embryos. Finally, taking antibiotics prophylactically was a form of genocide against the *jivās* in the wife's body. They abandoned further fertility treatments opting instead to take their chances with natural conception.

Questions for reflection

1. Is it possible to undergo IVF without forming an emotional attachment to the embryos created?

2. Could the wife have requested to proceed with the egg retrieval and refuse to take the antibiotics?
3. Would donating the embryos for scientific research not be for the greater good, even if it is an act of violence to destroy them?

Submitted by Whitny Braun de Lobatón

Glossary

Ācārya A spiritual preceptor; the head of a monastic order.
Ahiṁsā Non-violence; the chief of the five vows of the *vratas*.
Digambara Jain sect; translates as "sky-clad"; *Digambara* Jain male ascetics are nude.
Hiṁsā Violence.
Jina An omniscient person; a conqueror.
Jivā Soul; one of the five basic substances that make up the matter of the universe.
Karma 1. Action 2. Karma-matter or particles of Karma *Pudgala Vargaṇā* 3. Karmic encumbrance earned through one's mental, vocal, or physical activities.
Kevalin One who is omniscient.
Mokṣa Emancipation; Liberation.
Sādhu Monk.
Sādvī Nun.
Sallekhanā External and internal penance to weaken the body and passions before undertaking the practice of *Samādhimaraṇa*.
Samādhi The state of equanimity of mind or that of being peaceful, calm, and tranquil; psychic disposition of spiritual peace.
Saṁsāra The world of transmigration; the process of birth, death, and rebirth.
Santhārā 1. Literally, the grass bed on which the *kṣapaka* lies for his end practice. 2. Metaphorically, the practice of *Samādhimaraṇa*.
Siddha An emancipated soul.
Śramanic The religious traditions which do not believe in a supreme deity such as Jainism and Buddhism, unlike Hinduism which believes in a supreme divinity over the universe and is thus Bhramanic.
Śvetāmbara Jain sect; translates as "white clad."
Tīrthaṅkara The supreme religious leaders of Jainism; "Fordmaker."

Bibliography

Ācharanga Sutra (1996) Book 1, lecture 4, lesson 1, in Fox, MW. *The Boundless Circle: Caring for Creatures and Creation* (H. Jacobi, Trans.).
Baya, DS. (2006) "Relevance of Sallekhana in Today's Society and Euthanasia." Conference paper delivered at the International Summer School for Jain Studies, Jaipur, India.
Baya, DS. (2007) *Death with Eqaunimity: The Pursuit of Immortality*. Jaipur: Prakrit Bharati Academy.
Beauchamp, TL. (2003) "Methods and Principles in Biomedical Ethics," *Journal of Medical Ethics*, 29(5): 268–274.
Beauchamp, T., and Childress, J. (2001) *Principles of Biomedical Ethics*, 5th ed. New York: Oxford University Press.
Bhadrabahu. (1973) *Daśavaikālika Sūtra* (E. Leumann, Trans.). Motilal Banarsidass.

Bouvia v Superior Court, 179 Cal. App. 3d 1127, 1135-1136, 225 Cal. Rptr. 297. (Ct. App. 1986), review denied (Cal. June 5, 1986) and Bouvia v County of Los Angeles, 195 Cal. App. 3d 1075, 1080, 241 Cal. Rptr. 239 (1987).

Census of India (2011) *Census of India: Religion*. New Delhi, India: Registrat General & Census Commisioner of India. https://censusindia.gov.in/census.website/

Chapple, CK. (1993) *Nonviolence to Animals, Earth and Self in Asian Traditions*. New York: SUNY.

Cohan, JA. (2006) "Judicial Enforcement of Lifesaving Treatment for Unwilling Patients," *Creighton Law Review*, 39(4): 855.

Dundas, P. (2002) *The Jains. The Library of Religious Beliefs and Practices*. London: Routledge.

Ganzini, L., and Goy, ER. (2003) "Nurses' Experiences with Hospice Patients who Refuse Food and Fluids to Hasten Death," *New England Journal of Medicine*, 349(4): 359.

Glasenapp, H. von (1999) *Jainism: An Indian Religion of Salvation*. New Delhi, India: Motilal Banarsidass Publishers.

Jain, JP. (1999) *Religion and Culture of the Jains*. New Delhi: Bharatiya Jnanpith.

Jain, VK. (2018) *Ācārya Umāsvāmī's Tattvārthasūtra – With Explanation in English from Ācārya Pūjyapāda's Sarvārthasiddhi*. Vikalp Printers.

Jaini, PS. (1998) *The Jaina Path of Purification*. New Delhi, India: Motilal Banarsidass Publishers.

Jñātādharmakathāṅga sūtra: Pañcama Gaṇadhara Bhagavatsudharma-Svāmi-praṇīta ṣaṣṭha Aṅga: mūlapāṭha, Hindī anuvāda, vivecana, pariśiṣṭa yukta (1981) (Ś. Bhārilla, Trans.). Śrī Āgamaprakāśana-Samiti.

Kapur, D. (2010) *Diaspora, Development, and Democracy: The Domestic Impact of International Migration from India*. Princeton: Princeton University Press.

Kelting, MW. (2003) "Good Wives, Family Protectors: Writing Jain Laywomen's Memorials," *Journal of the American Academy of Religion*, 71(3): 640.

Keown, D. (1999) "Suicide, Assisted Suicide and Euthanasia: A Buddhist Perspective," *Journal of Law and Religion*, 13(2): 385–405.

Laidlaw, J. (2005) "A Life Worth Leaving: Fasting to Death as Telos of a Jain Religious Life," *Economy & Society*, 34(2): 178–199.

Lee, JHX. (2010) *Encyclopedia of Asian American Folklore and Folklife*. ABC-CLIO.

Mṛtyu Mahotsava (2010) (P. Rele, Trans.; Vol. 38). Hindi Grantha Karyalaya.

Settar, S. (2017) *Pursuing Death: Philosophy and Practice of Voluntary Termination of Life*, 2nd ed. Primus Books.

Shah, JB. (ed.) (2000) *Pt Sukhlalji's Commentary on Tattvartha Sutra of Vacaka Umasvati*, 2nd ed. Ahmedabad, India: L.D. Institute of Indology.

Sogani, KC. (2005) *Jainism: Ethico – Special Perspective*. Rajasthan: Jaina Vidya Samsthana.

Suriji, K. (2022) *Atur Pratyakhyan Sutra*. Sanmarg Prakashan.

Talbot, NA. (1983) "The Position of the Christian Science Church," *New England Journal of Medicine*, 39(26): 1641–1644.

Thomas, G. (2019) *Jain Community: Contribution to the UK*. United Kingdom Parliament House of Commons, Hansard. 659. https://hansard.parliament.uk/commons/2019-05-01/debates/93A69D0F-11C9-4428-857E-097031BC4B98/JainCommunityContributionToTheUK

Tukol, TK. (1976) *Sallekhana Is Not Suicide*. Ahmedabad, India: L.D. Institute of Indology.

Vallely, A. (2002) *Guardians of the Transcendent: An Ethnography of a Jain Ascetic Community*. Toronto: University of Toronto Press.

Wiltshire, MG. (1987) "The "Suicide" Problem in the Pali Cannon," *Journal of the International Association of Buddhist Studies*, 6(2): 124–140.

8 Chinese religions

Kwang-Hee Park

To be able under all circumstances to practice five things constitutes perfect virtue; these five things are gravity, generosity of soul, sincerity, earnestness, and kindness.

(*Confucian Analects* 1971: 112)

Manifest plainness, embrace simplicity, reduce selfishness, have few desires.

(*Lao Tzu* 1963)

Introduction

Chinese religion is a diverse and complex system of traditions that were developed throughout 2,000 years. Confucianism, Taoism, Buddhism, and popular folk religions are the four main traditions that have formulated the core of Chinese thought, cosmology, religious beliefs, and practice. Confucianism served as an ordering ethical principle to shape Chinese social roles and responsibilities. As a mystical religio-philosophical tradition, Taoism pursued longevity in interaction with nature. Buddhism, though a foreign import, expanded and deepened traditional religious beliefs and spiritual practices. The popular folk religions embraced diverse aspects of Taoism, Buddhism, and Confucianism and provided a practical guideline to promote prosperity and happiness in this world. Chinese religion is composed of practical and mysterious traditions that laid the foundation to create relational harmony between heaven and earth, between human beings and nature, and between the past and the present.

This chapter explores the beliefs and practices of traditional Chinese religion, primarily focusing on Confucianism and Taoism as indigenous traditions that influenced the formation of unique Chinese health beliefs and practices. In addition to these matters, the chapter introduces Chinese medicine as the integration of Chinese health beliefs and health practices and its clinical cautions. The practice of Chinese medicine in China and Taiwan is different from that of Traditional Chinese Medicine (TCM) in the United States. There is a limitation in the scope of practice of TCM in the United States compared to China or Taiwan.

Demographics

Traditional Chinese religions – Confucianism, Taoism, universism (a natural philosophy), divination practice, and Buddhist elements – are widely practiced in 60 countries around

DOI: 10.4324/9781003288862-8

the world with more than 225 million adherents. According to Pew Global Attitudes Project conducted in 2006, 31 percent of the population in China considers religion to be important in their lives. It is interesting to note that the 2005 survey finds that approximately three out of five Chinese believe in some form of supernatural phenomena associated with Confucianism and folk religion, such as fortune and fate, Jade Emperor, immortal souls, and ghosts. This suggests that popular religion may have permeated Chinese religious beliefs more than religious affiliation (Pew Forum on Religion and Public Life 2008).

According to figures from 2016, there are 1.4 billion inhabitants in China of whom hundreds of millions engage in diverse religious beliefs and practices. There are five official religions recognized by the Chinese government. These are Buddhism, Taoism, Islam, Catholicism, and Protestantism. The US government estimates that there are 657 million Chinese who follow some religion, including 250 million Buddhists, 70 million Christians, 25 million Muslims, 301 million observers of folk religions, and 10 million observers of other faiths, including Taoism (US State Department 2016). The government-sanctioned Taoist Association reports that there are more than 25,000 Taoist priests and nuns, 1,500 Taoist temples, and two Taoist schools. There are hundreds of millions of citizens who practice traditional folk religions (worship of local gods, heroes, and ancestors) which are often blended with Taoism, Buddhism, or ethnic minority cultural practices (US State Department 2007). In Taiwan, the Taoist population is, proportionally, larger than in mainland China. More than 80 percent of the Taiwanese people practice traditional Chinese folk religions (including also shamanism, animism, and ghost worship). Self-described spiritual practice is also popular. The sect movement of *Falun Gong* still holds its popularity, with approximately 2.1 million adherents, in spite of the Taiwanese government's oppression of the sect in 1999 (US State Department 2021a).

Even though Confucianism and Taoism lost their status as national religions, their ethical influence remains strong in East Asian countries, including Korea, Japan, and much of southeast Asia, with approximately 5.9 million adherents (US State Department 2021b). Taoism is practiced in the US by approximately 30,000 followers and approximately 2,000 in Canada. Taoism has enriched European and Asian cultures by introducing teachings of the Taoist classic text of *Tao Te Ching*, and promoting a holistic lifestyle and health practice that includes Chinese diet, art, martial arts, Qi-gong, and Chinese medicine (Smith 1986: 119).

History

Early Chinese religion originated from centuries of village agricultural life beginning in the eleventh century BCE. From early times, the Chinese believed in the existence of multiple gods and spirits in nature, gods of heaven and earth, and evil spirits (called *kuei*). They practiced ancestor worship, religious sacrifice, and offerings. During the Shang dynasty (1500–1040 BCE), the polytheistic and animistic religious beliefs were unified into a concept of a supreme God (*Shang Ti*) who was above all other gods and spirits, controlling human destiny on earth according to human deeds. Later, during the Zhou dynasty (770–200 BCE), the concept *Tian* or heaven developed, which controlled the spirits of the dead and bestowed "the mandate of Heaven" on individuals and worthy rulers. Additionally, ancestor worship, grave burial, and oracle bones for divination were introduced as religious practices (Oldstone-Moore 2003: 204).

The patriarchal and hierarchical feudal system of the Shang and Zhou dynasties was challenged by external invasions and subsequent appearances of new societal classes. Warlords, merchants, and serfs replaced the existing aristocratic class system. The feudal world fell apart. In search of solutions to the social and political instability, many Chinese philosophical schools sprang forth (400–300 BCE). These philosophical schools proposed distinctive concepts in order to bring peace and social stability. Confucianism and Taoism were two prominent philosophical schools. Confucius (551–479 BCE) proposed a strong and centralized government based on moral principles. Taoism, based on the philosophy of Lao-Tzu, favored no government at all (Hopfe 2007: 169). During the Han dynasty (220 BCE–206 CE), the teachings of Confucius won the argument with the Chinese imperial bureaucratic system consolidated through civil service examinations based on the texts and teachings of Confucius. Temples were built to honor Confucius. This bureaucratic society ran the country with Confucian values until the collapse of the Han dynasty.

Taoism opposed the morality-oriented government. Built on the philosophical theories of Lao-Tzu (sixth century BCE) and Chuang-Tzu (fourth century BCE), Taoism claimed that people should follow the natural and eternal way of the universe, *Tao*, not human principles. Philosophical Taoism was influenced by two sect movements: the Yellow Turbans (184–215 CE) and the Way of the Celestial Masters, sometimes referred to as the Way of Five Bushels of Rice (200–300 CE). The Yellow Turbans worshipped a mother goddess, Xi-wang-mu, the "Queen Mother of the West," who was believed to grant immortal life to those who chant her name (Overmyer 1986: 27–31). The Way of the Celestial Masters was initiated by Chang Tao-ling (34–156 CE), the founder and first leader of organized Taoism, who spread it to the public by introducing healing practices such as exorcism. Celestial Masters were exposed to mystical experiences and alchemy. They gradually established a religious system that included various rituals and chanting. The two sects laid the foundation upon which Taoism would be consolidated into an organized religion (Unschuld 1985: 39).

The traditional religions – Confucianism and Taoism – were colored by Buddhism, which was introduced from India to China in the third century CE. Buddhism introduced a complex Indian cosmology and the concept of universal salvation. The collapse of the Han dynasty in 206 CE allowed people freedom to choose their own religion and religious practice. Buddhists' ability to contextualize their faith (600–700 CE) enabled them to spread their influence. In the process, they developed the new concept of Pure Land in the afterlife and a new method of meditation called *chan* (*zen* in Japan). Pure Land Buddhism attracted a wide range of people and met needs in uncertain times with its devotional practices and promise of rebirth in a future world. Chan Buddhism resonated with philosophical Taoism, sharing the quest for the true nature of reality. Taoists even incorporated Buddhist teachings and monastic lifestyles and encouraged celibacy in pursuing religious life by adopting a nunnery system (900–1000 CE). In spite of its efforts, Buddhism has always been identified as "a foreign religion" by the Chinese and suffered periods of persecutions under the Confucian majority (Oldstone-Moore 2003: 205–206).

After its decline, Confucianism was revived during the Song dynasty (960–1279 CE) and spread its influence beyond China into Korea, Vietnam, and Japan. This period is called "the second great wave of revival" in Confucianism (Berthrong 2003: 26). When China was reunified under the Chin Dynasty (1115–1234 CE), Confucian philosophy was thriving again, having developed into a new form that has come to be known as neo-Confucianism. Chu Hsi (1130–1200 CE), the founder of neo-Confucianism, developed a complex belief combining Confucian morality with Buddhist meditation. He claimed that all things, including human nature, have an ordering principle, *li*, which is the source to shape the vital material *ch'i*. Humans must cultivate themselves in order to understand the underlying principle of *li* (Overmyer 1986: 48–51).

Reliance on the impersonal principle (*li*) in neo-Confucianism, however, led many educated people to search for more personal and emotional gods and religious experience. Popular religious practices and activities such as shamanism, veneration of ancestors, divination, belief in ghosts and demons, and exorcisms began to rise again. This is known as the Chinese folk religion, which combined diverse aspects of major concerns of the three religious traditions, but without a systematic belief system. Popular folk religion dealt with the worldly and practical issues such as longevity, prosperity, domestic harmony, continuing the family line by bearing children, and protection from disaster. While Confucians rebuked popular religious practices, Buddhist and Taoist priests went close to the people by conducting various folk rituals (Overmyer 1986: 48–51).

Since then, Confucianism, Taoism, Buddhism, and folk religion have blended and may simply be referred to as Chinese religion. New religions (Islam, Christianity) were introduced to China during the Ch'ing dynasty (1644–1912 CE). Under the Cultural Revolution (1966–1976 CE), however, all religions in China were suppressed and violent actions were taken against religious practitioners. Folk religions, Confucian temples, and even Confucius' birthplace were destroyed; Taoists shrines, altars, tablets, and relics were purged. With the death of the communist leader Mao Zedang, the Chinese government reintroduced religious freedom and allowed religious activities, writings, and clergy – albeit subject to government sanctions. Centers for religious studies were re-established in universities. The movement to restore Confucian teachings dating back to 1503 began to rise again. In Taiwan, on the other hand, popular Chinese folk religion and Taoism have long flourished with very few restrictions. On the whole, the four streams of the Chinese religion are thriving once again in Chinese society (Hopfe 2007: 177–187; Meulenbeld 2019).

Beliefs and practices

General

The diverse and complex beliefs in Chinese religion are deeply rooted in ancient Chinese cosmology as described in the classic text, the *I-Ching*. In Chinese cosmology, the world consists of both *yin* and *yang*, strength and weakness, health and sickness, success and failure, joy and sorrow. These polarities are not opposites. Nature embraces both. Nature maintains the two opposites and keeps them in tension. Hence any effort to logically analyze Nature ends with the analyzing person self-uprooting from Nature. When we seek to eliminate what we perceive as the negative aspect, we interfere with a complex system of relationships that we do not understand. The Chinese believed that *ch'i* was the vital substance that made up everything in the universe. *Ch'i* was thought to be manifested into *yin* and *yang* (the two complementary forces of the universe) and into five elements (metal, wood, water, fire, and earth) as the basic materials on the earth. Through *ch'i*, all things in the universe were co-related, interfused, and intermingled. There was interaction between heaven and earth, human beings and nature, and *yin* and *yang*. Ancient

Chinese saw reality as constantly changing and transforming in the interaction between *yin* and *yang* and among the five elements consisting of wood, fire, earth, metal, and water. Thus, existence in the universe could not be just a well-ordered static condition but the perpetual activity of creating a harmonized unity. The concept of harmony is the center of Chinese thought and is the common theme of Confucianism and Taoism (Chan 1963: 244–245).

Confucianism centered on creating social harmony on the basis of virtues. Confucius (551–479 BCE) studied classics, rituals, poems, and legend in order to restore peace and order in society. He realized the importance of ethical principles that can be applied to everyone. There are basic virtues that Confucius promoted. These are *jen* (benevolence to humanity), *li* (rites, traditional ceremonies, and formal patterns of conduct), and *chun-tzu* (superior person). *Jen* served as an inner ethical commitment and responsibility of the rulers to create a good government for their people. Confucius taught in his classic *Analects* that the inward power of empathy and compassion for others is the basis of morality. This should be expressed in daily life through *li* (courtesy). For Confucius, *jen* and *li* were two golden ethical standards that should be expressed in the form of virtues through the five basic human relationships (Hopfe 2007: 181).

The five basic human relationships, according to Confucianism, are the foundation of a morally principled, well-ordered, and harmonious society. These relationships exist between the paradigmatic father and son in which father has to behave kindly to his son and the son respects the father in filial piety. The relationships extend to elder brother (gentility) and younger brother (humility); husband (righteous behavior) and wife (obedience); elders (consideration) and juniors (deference); and rulers (benevolence) and subjects (loyalty). Confucians believe that family relationships and the virtue of filial piety (*hsiao*) among the five basic human relationships is the foundation to bond the family and community, thereby ultimately harmonizing and transforming society and cosmos (Hopfe 2007: 181).

A Confucian virtue-based harmonious society can be achieved through education and self-cultivation. Self-cultivation is the process to become an authentic person who is honest to self and loyal to others. The individual can expand and deepen communal action for humanity through education and self-discipline. Confucius called the fully developed moral self "superior person" or "gentleman" (*chun-tzu*). The gentleman is a man of *jen*, a harmonized self, which is expressed in appropriate moral conduct or courtesy (*li*) in social relationships. *Jen* and *li* are manifested in loving one another and practicing respect and courtesy toward one another. They are the inner moral core that motivates and guides a person to pursue the universal moral law of *Tao*, the foundation of the socio-political order of society. This is what Confucius calls respecting *t'ien-ming* (the mandate of heaven), which both the ruler and people must respect as the first principle. It is "the Way" (*Tao*) of heaven and the principle (*li*) of heaven or nature. Confucius' teaching of harmony claims that "human beings can make the Way (*Tao*) rather than the Way can make human beings great" (Chan 1963: 15–16; Meulenbeld 2019).

On the contrary, Taoism views the universe as being operated by *Tao*, which they understand as the mysterious way of the universe. The tradition of philosophical Taoism dates back to Lao-Tzu (sixth century BCE), the legendary founder of Taoism. He served the imperial bureaucracy and promoted a laissez-faire theory of government. His *Tao Te Ching* is the classic text of Taoism, which is composed of a short text with only 5,000 words. Taoists believe that everything in the universe (human knowledge, achievements, education, and morality) is transient and temporary and will decay. Nothing is to be viewed more precious than life itself on earth, thus enriching and prolonging life should be a person's primary concern. The best way of enriching an individual's life is to live in perfect harmony with *Tao*, the source and origin of all life, which, as the first cause, existed even before *yin* and *yang*, and heaven and earth (Hopfe 2007: 172).

According to Lao Tzu, the Tao is what it is. The recurring problems within the society stem from our discontent with what is. Emerging from this discontent are categories that we create for ourselves in order to strive for something we construct as better. It is this discontent in the very first place that is the cause for us to depart from the Tao. To return to the Tao is to follow the natural state through human's non-intervention, be able to embrace what is because that is the natural way of *Tao*. The individual has to take on a non-active, non-purposive state in order to access the *ch'i* (breath or life energy) of *Tao*, which is manifested as *yin* and *yang*, the two forces of nature. *Ch'i* forms and dissolves all things in the universe. Non-interference (*wu-wei*) is the best way that the individual can be tuned to and be harmonized with *Tao*, thereby accessing the maximum of *ch'i* for a healthy and long life, even achieving immortality. "Vitalizing Taoists" who utilized *ch'i* attempted to remove obstructions in the flow of *ch'i* and maximize it through breathing techniques and practicing immortality (a health and spiritual practice that aims at cultivating inner and outer self to achieve spiritual immortality). The practice of immortality was later reinforced by religious Taoists who claimed divine revelations for immortality and led temple worship services, rituals, exorcisms, and healings for spiritual communities. Taoists pursue self-cultivation of *ch'i* and *yin-yang* balance in interaction with the harmonious relationship with the *Tao*. While Confucians pursue a harmonized self, based on self-cultivated virtues or moral principles, Taoists pursue a harmonized self, based on a simple, spontaneous (*tzu-jan*), and tranquil lifestyle (Smith 1986: 128–134; Kleeman 2017).

Both Confucians and Taoists aim at conserving *te* (virtue) as the goal of self-transformation. For Confucius, this *te* is a perfect moral state, a manifestation of the universal moral law of *Tao* (Unschuld 1985: 60–62). Taoists view that *te* is a simple and weak way to let nature flow and take its own course. It is not a passive withdrawal from reality or government, but a practical strategy to oppose the controlling morality-based government at the time. Taoists view that self-transformation can take place by pursuing a natural lifestyle following and nourishing one's own human nature, *Tao*, as well as enjoying and returning to nature (Chan 1963: 136–137). Chuang-Tzu explained that he himself harmonizes all things in the universe and transcends the self beyond the control of the government. As disparate as they are in their approaches, Confucianism and Taoism are in common pursuit of harmony with *Tao* in their core. The Confucian balanced self is achieved through harmonious human relationships in social settings, while the Taoist balanced self is pursued in harmonious interaction with nature.

Pursuit of a harmonious relationship with *Tao* in social settings and in the natural sphere was practiced through life events, religious activities, longevity, meditation, and seasonal occasions. Confucians' self-cultivating education was promoted through rituals that marked a series of life events. *Jiali*, a book of family rituals, describes the four basic Confucian rituals: capping (a coming of age ceremony for boys), wedding, funeral service, and ancestor worship (Yu 2002: 71–82). Ancestor worship was a central religious activity which carried from generation to generation reinforcing the core virtue of Confucianism: filial piety. Confucians believed that spirits of ancestors and of the dead have the power to influence the lives of the descendants by either blessing or cursing them. Ancestor worship is a religious and communal activity in which human beings and divinities exchange a meal or offerings (Overmyer 1986: 24; Meulenbeld 2019).

The Chinese medical ethical principle of "benevolence for all humanity" emphasizes the equality of all when providing treatment, regardless of gender, social status, age, etc. In the Chinese society, however, women's roles have been secondary to men in the domestic and public arena. Women developed a non-assertive self and sacrificed themselves for the sake of the harmony of the family. In medical practice, women have tended to hide their medical or family problems from outsiders in order not to bring shame or humiliation to the family. When the medical problems are related to contagious diseases, such as sexually transmitted diseases or HIV, women are more exposed to negative consequences (e.g., blame, physical violence, emotional torture, and abuse) from family and society. When men disclose sexually transmitted diseases, it is of less concern, even in cases of infection to other family members, due to the superior position that men hold in the family (Yang et al. 2006: 722). Thus, contrary to Confucian medical ethics, women today still face an unequal treatment in the patriarchal Chinese culture.

The Chinese have also taken seriously funeral rituals which were believed to send the deceased to a peaceful journey into the afterlife – a practice that shows a strong Buddhist influence. During the funeral ceremony, mourners throw dates on the coffin to ask the ancestors to bless their descendants with children. The Chinese believe strongly in the connection from the dead to the living and the past to the present. The harmonious relationship between them is considered to facilitate blessings for the living. The open coffin is placed in the main room of the house during the days of funeral rituals. During the services, food is offered to the spirit of the dead, and prayers are offered to gods for the deceased loved one's safe passage to the underworld. The appropriate gravesite for the deceased is often chosen through *feng-shui* (wind and water) to ensure a safe and peaceful place for the deceased and for the living to receive benevolence and blessings from ancestors. *Feng-shui* pursues the sacred power in the natural environment and a harmonious life within the natural order (Yang et al. 2006: 61–63; Chan & Chow 2017). In recent years, it has become popular even in the West as a method to access prosperity and harmony in the home, workplace, and the business world (Oldstone-Moore 2003: 223).

A variety of meditation techniques have grown out of these early alchemy techniques. All three Chinese traditions – Confucianism, Taoism, Buddhism – practice meditation. Confucians practice "quiet sitting" in order to reflect on Confucian teachings or meditate on patterns of order (*li*) to strengthen the moral order of society. *Chan* (*zen*) meditative Buddhist groups practice the emptying of the egocentric mind and thoughts in a support group atmosphere. Taoists employ meditative techniques to enhance a new awareness of the cosmic power within the practitioner's body (Overmyer 1986: 77–79). Taoist alchemy masters teach people through meditation to help them internalize the spiritual forces of *ch'i* (life energy), *shen* (spiritual consciousness), and *Tao* (Kirkland 2002: 178). The pursuit of harmony between the mind and the body is the basis of all meditation techniques.

The blended aspects of the Chinese traditions are broadly celebrated through seasonal events as well. The Pure and Bright Festival (early April) is the occasion when the descendants visit the graves of the ancestors. The boat races and rice cakes of the Dragon Boat Festival (June) celebrate the highest *yang* power on earth and the beginning of the *yin* power. During the Dragon Boat Festival, Taoists still practice exorcism and drive out evil spirits thought to cause diseases or harm among people. Buddhism has influenced the All Soul's Day (late August) as an occasion to release the souls of ancestors or wandering spirits from the underworld (the place where the souls that have not been reborn reside) through offerings. Finally, during the autumn Harvest Festival and winter holidays, ancestors, hero gods, or patron saints are worshipped through thanksgiving (Hopfe 2007: 185–186).

Health and disease

To follow the natural rhythm of *Tao* is the central thought that has formed the health belief of the Chinese. *Tao* is manifested in dynamic changes of the *yin-yang* energies, allotment of *ch'i*, and interaction of the five elements of water, fire, wood, metal, and earth. According to Taoists, humans and nature are mutually interdependent. Humans must conform to the natural rhythms of the universe in order to achieve health and longevity. Harmony between *yin* and *yang*, free flow of *ch'i*, and balance among the five elements are the three most important elements in understanding the Chinese concept of health and illness (Ni 1995: 17).

When there is harmony between *yin* and *yang* and among the five elements in the body, there is a natural flow of *ch'i*. The Chinese believed that *ch'i* is embedded in all existence, whether humans, trees, rocks, etc. *Ch'i* is part of the energy in the human body. As an allotment of *Tao*, *ch'i* is expressed in the *yin* and *yang* forces, balancing the interaction of the five elements (wood, fire, earth, metal, and water) that correspond with the human body, such as the heart (fire), the liver (wood), kidneys (water), the pancreas (earth), and the lungs (metal). Human body parts interact with nature through *ch'i*. When a person is attuned to the natural flow of *ch'i* in nature, she or he may become healthy. If the *ch'i* flow in the body is blocked by such "evils" as weather conditions (cold, hot, wind, damp, etc.), *ch'i* deficiency or excess, or emotional stress, disharmony of the *yin* and *yang* energies occurs, leading to a break in the nourishing cycle among the five elements and resulting in diseases and death. Death is the state of complete separation between the *yin* and *yang* energies (Hai et al., 2022).

In the Chinese view, the human body is a holistic microcosm that embraces *ch'i*, *yin*, and *yang*, and the five elements in interaction with the macrocosm of nature. This health concept is not just limited to the physical aspect of the human body but also includes psychological and spiritual elements in interaction with nature and the environment. A holistic concept of health under the influence of *Tao* (*ch'i*, *yin*, and *yang*, and the five elements) is applied to diverse health practices among the Chinese. Chinese medicine, meditation, exercise, and nutrition therapy are common health practices. These practices when held in balance promote a natural lifestyle that helps incline a person to the natural rhythm of *Tao*, which contributes ultimately to enhanced health and longevity.

Common tools in the practice of Chinese medicine include acupuncture, herbal practice, nutrition therapy, and exercise. Acupuncture emphasizes that *ch'i* in the body is circulated via 12 meridians or channels to nourish the five major organs (liver, heart, spleen, lungs, and kidneys) and other parts of the body. When *ch'i* is obstructed, it creates imbalance between the *yin* and *yang* energies in patterns of either excess or deficiency, hot or cold, or interior or exterior to the body. Disharmony between the *yin* and *yang* energies causes abnormality and disease. Thus, the goal of acupuncture treatment is to restore the balance of the *yin-yang* energy, hot and cold, exterior and interior, and deficiency and excess patterns in interaction with *Tao*. This *yin* and *yang* energy balance is believed to not only prevent diseases but also enhance the immune system (Bowman & Hui 2000: 1482).

Acupuncture is considered one of the most safe, effective, and low-cost healthcare modes, with few side effects. Apart from usual meridian-oriented acupuncture treatment, diverse forms and techniques of acupuncture treatments are practiced – such as ear, hand, and scalp acupunctures, electrical acupuncture, and acupuncture treatment based on different body constitutions (Maciocia 1989: 320–322). Aside from acupuncture, other traditional Chinese treatments include herb therapy, nutrition (food), moxibustion (heat therapy using mug wort herbs), cupping, and *gua-sha* therapy (scraping the skin) to enhance the *yin-yang* balance.

Health practices of the Chinese also include mind therapy or mind–body therapy. Meditation is a popular form of exercise to achieve a deeper state of self-awareness. This meditative process includes psychological, physiological, and spiritual disciplines in order to reach a higher state of consciousness and create a peaceful mind. Animating meditation or yoga promotes the inner self (Smith 1986: 130–131). Mind–body exercises are practiced in the form of martial arts both in China and elsewhere in the world, including the United States – such as *tai-chichuan* and *ch'i kung*. Many Chinese elderly engage in these arts early in the morning, combining breathing exercises with slow body movements. They also provide a social and environmental context where people get to know one another. Daily devotion to these arts strengthens the mind–body unit and promotes the circulation of *ch'i*. *Ch'i kung* is also a viable alternative exercise whenever there is a barrier to other forms of exercise – be it due to old age, physical disability, or slow physical rehabilitation. For stress-related diseases, it promotes physiological and psychological well-being in a relaxed, calm, and energized environment (Jouper et al. 2006: 949–957).

The Chinese worldview upholds a respect for life at its beginning and its end. Chinese medical ethics is greatly influenced by the core Confucian belief of benevolence toward all humanity. This universal ethical value is practiced in order to venerate and respect human life. Regardless of social class, family background, age, or sex, caregivers are called to love people and sustain and prolong life (Confucianism) over accepting death as a natural process (Taoism) (Jouper et al. 2006: 949–957).

Births – and male births in particular – are welcomed in Chinese society. Therefore, the Chinese cultural attitude toward abortion is generally negative, particularly in the case of male fetuses. The Confucian principle of filial piety encourages reproduction, especially of male offspring, as a responsibility to one's parents. The Confucian valuation of life is further strengthened by the Buddhist teaching of compassion and prohibition against killing any living beings. Thus, life is always viewed as precious and the taking of a life is something to be cautiously dealt with. At the same time, Chinese women are allowed to take initiative in making a decision on abortion when there is a high risk of hereditary or genetic disability (Baoqi & Macer 2005: 27).

Death and dying

The Chinese have understood death and dying as part of life. Both Taoism and Confucianism view that life comes from the mother, earth, and *yin* and returns to the father, heaven, and *yang*. Death and dying is simply a natural flow of life to return to its origin – *Tao*, where life starts. Even though Confucius' primary focus was on present life and human beings on earth, he dealt with the issues of death and spirits with sensitivity (Wei-ming 1986: 55–70). Ancestor worship and funeral rituals have strengthened the continuum of time between the dead and the living and between the past and the present. Taoists' understanding of death is similar to that of Confucians. Life and death are two complementary aspects of reality, the unchanging *Tao*; thus, death is the change from being to non-being, from *yang* to *yin*. Death is considered to have equal value to life, thus death should not be feared. A contemporary Chinese thanatologist summarizes the understanding of the Chinese attitude toward life and death as "*zhong sheng an si,*" which means "respecting life seriously and accepting death peacefully." Confucians accept death with a willingness to preserve virtue and dignity, thus human beings should not be afraid of death. Humans can make a choice to die rather than making a non-virtuous effort to preserve life. Buddhists believe that death is a process of rebirth on the passage to nirvana (Tse et al. 2003: 339–343: Chan & Chow 2017). When life on earth comes to its end, the Chinese perceive death as natural, even as an extension of life. The dying person feels safe and has a sense of belonging at home. Therefore, Chinese patients with terminal cancer usually wish to die in their own homes rather than in a hospital (Chen 2001: 270–273).

Withdrawing life support is still a difficult issue in China. When it is practiced in the settings of healthcare in the West, it should be handled with great sensitivity. It may be an offensive or reluctant issue for Chinese patients (Klessig 1992: 316–322). The centuries-long influence of traditional religious beliefs affects the issue of euthanasia. Buddhists view killing or shortening life as an evil act which will be punished in a subsequent life. The Chinese ethical principle of respect for life, influenced by Confucianism and Taoism, seeks to avoid advancing the process of death and dying. The Confucian ethical value of filial piety promotes keeping parents alive as long as possible. Despite opposition to euthanasia among most lawyers in China, healthcare professionals and the public are paying more attention to the issue of quality of life for patients, thus passive euthanasia is being gradually accepted in China (Li & Chou 1997: 809, 243–248; Li 2013). The awareness of cultural differences in accepting and practicing death and dying will allow health practitioners to support end-of-life processes of Chinese patients with sensitivity.

Table 8.1 Dos and don'ts

Dos	Don'ts
1. Grant the family as much influence and involvement as possible.	1. Do not marginalize the family.
2. If need be, serve as a patient advocate if the possibility of family manipulation shows itself.	2. Do not be surprised at the presence of benevolent deception with terminally ill patients.
3. Recognize that medical decisions are not placed solely in the hands of the patient and may be solely in the hands of the family.	3. Do not bring up the topic of organ donation.
4. Know that more traditional Chinese may be reluctant to discuss advance directives.	4. Do not speak openly about death as some believe that to do so may hasten death.
5. Understand that most traditional Chinese will strongly desire to die at home.	5. Do not hold on to prejudice against Traditional Chinese Medicine, which is widely practiced in Chinese American communities.
	6. Do not openly discuss mental disorder/disease and psychiatric services.

Conclusion

Confucianism, Taoism, Buddhism, and popular folk religions have combined in the Chinese experience to form a diverse and complex system of traditions. Confucianism helped shape Chinese social roles and responsibilities. Taoism's mystical religio-philosophical tradition has pursued longevity in interaction with nature. Buddhism expanded and deepened traditional religious beliefs and spiritual practices. Popular folk religions embraced diverse aspects of each of these traditions and provided practical guidelines for daily life. Chinese religion is composed of practical and mystical traditions that have laid the foundation to create relational harmony between heaven and earth, between human beings and nature, and between the past and the present.

Case study #1

An unmarried 21-year-old Chinese American male lay in a hospital following a motor-cycle accident. His driver's license indicated his registration as an organ donor. Verified as brain dead, his body on a mechanical ventilator awaited the procurement of transplant-able body organs. As the legal owners of the deceased man's body, his parents agreed to the organ procurement but also requested that his sperm be extracted and frozen with the aim of producing a male child with a surrogate. His parents say he wanted a family and explain that in Chinese culture their family name is carried on through the male line.

It is generally accepted practice for hospitals and physicians to support postmortem sperm retrieval. But the guidelines typically state that parental requests do not necessarily have to be honored.

The hospital administration and the medical staff indicate a willingness to accede to the parents' request but insist on a court order, given the rarity of the request. A local county judge rules in favor of the parents' urgent request for sperm retrieval. Whether or not his parents (the potential child's grandparents) will be allowed to engage/employ a surrogate to carry their child/grandchild remains unclear. A staff urologist extracts their son's still viable sperm.

Questions for reflection

1. Given the absence of any written documentation of the son's desires, what weight should be given to the parents' claim that the deceased son, out of filial loyalty, would agree with their intention to raise a child conceived with his sperm and thus preserve the family name?
2. Can the parents' plan be ethically justified using the principle of respect for autonomy?
3. The judge merely granted permission for the collection of sperm. Should the parents be granted legal permission to proceed with their plan for artificial insemination with the aid of a surrogate? If so, with what constraints? If not, on what grounds?

Submitted by Ernest J. Bursey

Case study #2

Recently, our institution formed a "sister hospital" relationship with a healthcare organ-ization in China. As the nurse educator for my surgical rehab unit, I was selected to go to

China as part of a clinical education team that would focus on issues at the intersection of bioethics and religion.

As China has opened up to more foreign people living there, religion and associated ideas of morality have subsequently become more important. Of course, in the US, religion and abortion is a moral issue, so I naturally thought I would include the topic of abortion in my course at the sister hospital. While developing my course, however, I asked the nurse educator there to review my session goals, and I was surprised when she advised me not to include abortion in my material.

In the past, China's "one child policy" meant that forced abortions became routine. Apparently, women of all faiths in China almost surely have had an abortion at some point. Thus, per my educator partner in China, abortion was not a moral issue, and so it did not belong in a hospital ethics course.

Questions for reflection

1. What religious traditions consider abortion a moral issue?
2. If lots of religious people have undergone abortions in China, should that automatically take it off a list of issues to be addressed in a hospital ethics course?
3. If the government forces someone to get an abortion and it is not a personal choice, does that remove the moral onus often associated with it?
4. If and when the issue of choice is taken off the table, what other moral issues emerge surrounding abortion in Chinese life and culture?

*Submitted by Mark F. Carr

Glossary

Ch'I Implies "breath of life" or "life energy," derived from Tao. In Chinese medicine, *ch'i* is the essence that maintains the functions of the body.

Chun-tzu The name of the religious leaders who taught and practiced the five virtues of self-respect, generosity, sincerity, persistence, and benevolence to others.

Jen Translated as "benevolence for all humanity." *Jen* in Confucianism is compared to the Golden Rule in Christianity: "Do not do to others what you would not like them to do to you" (Analects 15:23).

Li Translated as "propriety, reverence, courtesy, and ritual." *Li* implies a person's right moral conduct that is expressed through ceremony, rites, and courtesy in the human relationships.

Tao The origin of *Tao* is mysterious. It may be translated as the Path. But it is the Path that cannot be named or conceptualized. It encompasses everything. *Tao* is characterized as ultimate transcendent reality that guides the way of human life.

Wu-wei Means literally "inaction." It implies "pure effectiveness" in Taoism and is often used to refer to a spontaneous act that emerges from harmony with the self and reality.

Yin and yang The two complementary forces of the universe. *Yin* symbolizes night, dark, soft, cold, stillness, and feminine. *Yang* represents day, bright, warm, movement, and masculine. All phenomena in the universe are the expression of the interaction between *yin* and *yang*. These two forces are opposite but mutually interacting and inter-transforming.

Bibliography

Baoqi, S., and Macer, DRJ. (2005) "A Sense of Autonomy is Preserved Under Chinese Reproductive Policies," *New Genetics and Society*, 24(1): 15–29.

Berthrong, J. (2003) "Boston: The Third Wave of Global Confucianism," *Journal of Ecumenical Studies*, 40(1–2): 26.

Bowman, KW., and Hui, EC. (2000) "Bioethics for Clinicians: 20, Chinese Bioethics," *Canadian Medical Association Journal*, 163(11): 1481–1485.

Chan, S., and Chow, A. (2017) "A Cultural Sociological Review of Chinese Funeral Rituals," in Thompson, R and Cox, G. (eds) *Handbook of the Sociology of Death, Grief, and Bereavement: A Guide to Theory and Practice* (pp. 351–364). New York: Routledge.

Chan, W. (1963) *A Source Book in Chinese Philosophy*. New Jersey: Princeton University Press.

Chen, Y. (2001) "Chinese Values, Health and Nursing," *Journal of Advanced Nursing*, 36(2): 270–273.

Confucian Analects: The Great Learning, and The Doctrine of the Mean (1971) (J. Legge, Trans.). http://wengu.tartarie.com/wg/wengu.php?l=Lunyu&no=453

Hai, H., Wee, K., and Soh, SB. (2022) *Chinese Medicine for Health: Holistic Healing, Inner Harmony and Herbal Recipes*. Singapore: WSPC. https://doi.org/10.1142/13050

Hopfe, LM. (2007) *Religions of the World*, revised by MR. Woodward, 10th ed. Upper Saddle River, NJ: Pearson/Prentice Hall.

Jouper, J., Hassmén, P., and Johansson, M. (2006) "*Qi-gong* Exercise with Concentration Practice Increases Health," *American Journal of Chinese Medicine*, 34(6): 949–957.

Kirkland, R. (2002) "The History of Taoism: A New Outline," *Journal of Chinese Religions*, 30: 178–183.

Kleeman, T. (2017) "Daoism and Popular Religion in Imperial Chin," *Oxford Research Encyclopedia of Asian History*. https://oxfordre.com/asianhistory/view/10.1093/acrefore/9780190277727.001.0001/acrefore-9780190277727-e-207.

Klessig, J. (1992) "The Effect of Values and Culture on Life-Support Decisions," *The Western Journal of Medicine*, 157(3): 316–322.

Lao Tzu (1963) *The Tao Te Ching*. (Wing Tsit Chan, Trans.). The Terebess Asia Online. https://terebess.hu/english/tao/chan.html#Kap19

Li, LB. (2013) "Clinical Review: Ethics and End-of-Life Care for Critically Ill Patients in China," *Critical Care*, 17(6): 244. https://doi.org/10.1186/cc13140

Li, S., and Chou, JL. (1997) "Communication with the Cancer Patient in China," *Annual of the New York Academy of Science*, 809: 243–248.

Maciocia, G. (1989) *A Comprehensive Text for Acupuncturists and Herbalists*. Oxford: Churchill Livingstone.

Meulenbeld, M. (2019) "Confucianism, Daoism, Buddhism, and Chinese Popular Religion," *Oxford Research Encyclopaedia*. https://doi.org/10.1093/acrefore/9780190277727.013.126

Ni, M. (1995) "The Manifestation of *Yin* and *Yang* from the Macrocosm to the Microcosm," in *The Yellow Emperor's Classic of Medicine: A New Translation of the Neijing Suwen with Commentary* (pp. 13–16). Boston: Shambhala.

Oldstone-Moore, J. (2003) "Chinese Traditions," in Coogan, MD. (ed.) *World Religions: The Illustrated Guide* (pp. 200–235). London: Duncan Baird Publishers.

Overmyer, DL. (1986) *Religions of China: Religious Traditions of the World*. San Francisco: HarperCollins.

Pew Forum on Religion and Public Life (2008) "Religion in China on the eve of the 2008 Beijing Olympics." http://pewforum.org/docs/?DocID=301

Schwartz, BI. (1985) *The World of Thought in Ancient China*. Cambridge, MA: Harvard University Press.

Smith, H. (1986) *The Illustrated World's Religions: A Guide to our Wisdom Traditions*. San Francisco: HarperCollins.

Tse, CY., Chong, A., and Fok, SY. (2003) "Breaking Bad News: A Chinese Perspective," *Palliative Medicine*, 17(4): 339–343, quoted from the original Chinese edition by Zheng Xiaojiang (1994) *Philosophy of Death in the Chinese*, Taipei: Dong Da.

Unschuld, PU. (1985) *Medicine in China: A History of Ideas*. Los Angeles: University of California Press.

US State Department (2007) *Report on International Religious Freedom*. The Bureau of Democracy, Human Rights, and Labor Report. www.state.gov/j/drl/rls/irf/2007/

US State Department (2016) *International Religious Freedom Reports: China, Hong Kong, Macau, Tibet*. State.gov. www.state.gov/report/custom/e41aa7d9db/

US State Department (2021a) *International Religious Freedom Reports: Taiwan*. State.gov. www.state.gov/reports/2021-report-on-international-religious-freedom/taiwan/

US State Department (2021b) *International Religious Freedom Reports: China (Includes Tibet, Xinjian, Hong Kong and Macau)*. State.gov. www.state.gov/report/custom/24c46276d1/

Wei-ming, T. (1986) "The Confucian Tradition: A Confucian Perspective on Learning to Be Human," in Whaling, F. (ed.) *The World's Religious Traditions: Current Perspectives in Religious Studies* (pp. 55–70). New York: Crossroad.

Yang, H., Li, X., Stanton, B., Fang, X., Lin D., and Naar-King, S. (2006) "HIV-Related Knowledge, Stigma, and Willingness to Disclose: A Mediation Analysis," *AIDS Care*, 18(7): 61–63.

Yu, Z. (2002) "Confucian Education: A Moral Approach," *Religion East & West*, 2: 71–82.

9 Sikhism

Arvind Mandair

Ego is given to man as his disease. Disease affects all creatures that arise in the world except those who remain detached. Man is born in sickness, in sickness he wanders through birth after birth. Captive to disease he finds no rest, without the Guru sickness never stops.

(Adi Granth, as cited in Mandair 2013: 180)

Introduction

Sikhism refers to the way of life of those who call themselves Sikh, the way of life that embraces equality for all human beings and disapproves of every form of discrimination. Although the etymology of the word Sikh can be traced to the Sanskrit *sisya* or its Pali derivation *Sekkha*, the Punjabi term Sikh refers to the followers of Guru Nanak, his nine successors, and their teachings embodied in the Guru Granth Sahib or the sacred scripture of the Sikhs.

Demographics

The Sikh population worldwide is estimated at 20 million. Of these, 17 million Sikhs reside in India, with 14 million of them living in the Punjab region – the traditional Sikh homeland (US State Department 2018). Of the two million or so Sikhs who live outside India, comprising what is known as the Sikh diaspora, the majority are dispersed in countries such as Great Britain, the United States, Canada, East Africa, Malaysia, and Australia.

It is estimated that 500,000 Sikhs live in the United States, with about 100,000 of them living in California (Rosentiel 2012). Yuba City, CA., located 40 miles north of Sacramento, has the largest Sikh population in the country. There are 15,000 Sikhs living in and between Yuba City and Sacramento.

History

Sikhism originated in the Punjab region of Northwestern India during a time of Muslim–Hindu conflict. At this time a broadly aligned association of religious teachers known as the Sants were seeking to reconcile these two opposed socio-religious traditions. The Sants expressed their teachings in vernacular poetry and distinguished the belief that salvation is to be based on inner experience rather than personalized incarnations.

DOI: 10.4324/9781003288862-9

Although the teachings of Guru Nanak were broadly aligned with the Sants, his own mission emerged out of a direct experience of the divine initiated with the words *na koi Hindu, na koi Mussalman* (there is no Hindu, there is no Muslim) signaling a third way that was to become the *Nanak Panth* or the path of Nanak. The early community, which comprised those who chose to follow Nanak as their guru, was initially drawn largely from a Hindu background.

Nanak was born in 1469 (CE, and hereafter) in Talwandi, a village 40 miles from Lahore, and acclaimed by Muslims and Hindus alike as a future religious leader. Although he had received a formal education and held a post as a village accountant, Nanak's main preoccupation in his early life was with spiritual concerns and he preferred the company of saints and ascetics. Together with his closest associate, a Muslim bard named Mardana, Nanak organized regular nightly singing of devotional hymns, as well as going to bathe in a nearby river before daybreak. During one of these sessions, at age 30, Nanak underwent his first major mystical experience in which he received a calling to teach people a path of devotion to the divine Name. Shortly after this experience, Nanak embarked on a series of travels that took him eastwards to Banaras, Bengal, and Orissa, southward to Tamil Nadu and Sri Lanka, northward to Tibet, and finally west-ward to the Muslim regions going as far as Mecca, Medina, and Baghdad. In the final phase of his life at about the age of 50, Nanak founded a settlement at Kartarpur where he led a community of disciples instructing them in spiritual practice and study making *nam simaran* (remembrance of the Name) and *kirtan* (singing hymns of praise), regular features of devotion. At the same time, he insisted that his disciples remain fully involved in worldly affairs by doing practical labor (Nanak himself tended his own crops) while maintaining a regular family life.

Shortly before his death in 1539, at age 70, Guru Nanak's appointment of a successor not only inaugurated a two-centuries-long politico-spiritual lineage with each successor taking on the title guru, but also marked a break with prior Sant practice of not appointing spiritual successors. During the next two centuries, the early Sikh Panth (community) underwent significant expansion and development into a defined and disciplined order, with different steps taking place under successive gurus. The second guru, Angad (1504–1552), collected Nanak's hymns, developed the alphabetic script called Gurmukhi (lit-erally "from the guru's mouth"), and institutionalized the *langar* or communal kitchen to feed disciples who came to visit Nanak's *dharamsalas*, or rest house. Guru Amardas (1497–1574), the third guru, encouraged the observance of separate Sikh shrines, pil-grimage traditions, and festivals, as well as instituting the *manji* system of supervising distant congregations. The fourth guru, Ramdas (1534–1581), founded a new center called Ramdaspur (later named Amritsar) where he supervised the excavation of the sacred pool that later became the central site of Sikh pilgrimage. Guru Ramdas appointed *masands* or deputies to represent the guru's authority in his more dispersed congregations.

Sikhism became more firmly established under the fifth guru, Arjan (1563–1606). However, the increasing success and expansion of the Sikhs in Punjab at this time led to confrontation with the Mughal imperial authority under the Emperor Jahangir. Guru Arjan was accused of supporting a rebellion led by Jahangir's son, Amir Khusro. Charges of sedition were followed by imprisonment and finally execution in Lahore in 1606. Guru Arjan's martyrdom led to increased militarization and overt political involvement under his son and successor, the sixth guru, Hargobind (1595–1644), symbolized by his donning of two swords, one representing spiritual authority (*miri*), the other representing political authority (*piri*). Maintaining a small but effective army, Hargobind consciously prepared the Sikhs to resist wilful state oppression. Although confrontation receded during the tenure of his successor gurus, Har Rai and Har Krishan, they nevertheless maintained a similar style of leadership with a retinue of armed followers. It was the ninth guru, Tegh Bahadur (1621–1675), who again was forced to confront the increasingly restrictive policies of Jahangir's grandson, the Emperor Aurangzeb (1658–1707), which included enforcement of Islamic laws and taxes and the replacement of local Hindu temples by Muslim mosques. Guru Tegh Bahadur's active resistance against such policies, his public defense of Hindus' right to practice their religion freely, and his own refusal to accept Islam under pain of death led to his imprisonment and eventual execution in Chandni Chowk, one of Delhi's busiest markets, in 1675.

The Sikh Panth's involvement in political resistance came to a climax with the tenth guru, Gobind Singh (1666–1708). His best known contribution to the development of Sikhism was to redefine the very core of the Sikh Panth as a military-cum-spiritual order, the Khalsa (sovereign or free). According to tradition he called his followers to assemble for the Baisakhi festival in 1699 at Anandpur. There he called for five volunteers to pass a test of absolute loyalty. Those who passed the test, the so-called *panj piare* (Five Beloved Ones) were initiated into the new Khalsa order via a ceremonial rite called *khande ka pahul* (baptism of the double-edged sword), thus forming the nucleus of a sovereign, casteless community. Each member of the Khalsa order undertook to wear the five external symbols, or the five Ks (*kesh* – long, uncut hair; *kirpan* – short sword; *kangha* – comb; *kara* – steel bracelet; *kaccha* – breeches), to adhere to a formal code of conduct (*rahit*), and to relinquish family surnames with males assuming the name Singh (literally, lion) and females assuming the name Kaur (meaning princess), thereby removing sexual inequality whilst maintaining gender difference. The guru in turn received the same initiation from the *panj piare*, assuming the name Singh, signifying a merger of identities between the guru and disciple. Many thousands more accepted this initiation.

The creation of the Khalsa brought into existence a parallel but two-tier system within the developing Sikh community. On the one hand, there were the Khalsa Sikhs, namely, those who took initiation into the Khalsa had effectively agreed to mark their bodies in a particular way – specifically by not allowing bodily hair to be trimmed, and in the case of Sikh males, of wearing a turban to cover the long, uncut hair. On the other hand were the so-called *Sahajdhari* Sikhs (slow adopters), those who in every other way lived by the teachings of the Sikh gurus but had not undertaken formal initiation into the order of the Khalsa. During the eighteenth and early nineteenth centuries, the relationship between Khalsa and Sahajdhari Sikhs was a relatively fluid one such that individual families could claim to have members belonging to both groupings. However, this distinction became more pronounced in the late nineteenth and early twentieth centuries and especially with the formulation of the modern Sikh code of conduct in 1954. This new code of conduct helped to establish Khalsa Sikhs as a more or less "orthodox" component of the Sikh community.

The advent of British colonial rule not only marks the entry of Sikhism into Western modernity, but also the emergence of several reform movements attempting to revive a sense of religious identity at a time when most such traditions were considered to be sects of Hinduism. By far the most influential Sikh reformist movement was the Singh Sabha founded in 1883 under aristocratic patronage. Through its political functionary, the Chief Khalsa Diwan (CKD), a body set up in 1902 to jointly conduct its affairs, the Singh Sabha movement achieved the most successful reinterpretation of Sikhism adapted to modernity which has, until recently, exerted a hegemonic influence on Sikh self-consciousness. Their reformulation was based on the colonially inspired distinction between, on the one hand, a monotheistic-historical Sikhism centered on the authority of a clearly recognizable scripture and embodied by the Tat (authentic) Khalsa ideal, and on the other hand, a pantheistic ahistorical Hinduism. The leading Singh Sabha scholars redefined the doctrinal foundations of Sikhism in a way that would have been unimaginable only a few decades earlier. Under the banner of the Akali Dal, political successors to the Singh Sabha and the CKD, a campaign was launched in the early 1920s to wrest control of the Harimandar and other historical gurdwaras from the Mahants or traditional custodians, resulting in the Sikh Gurdwaras Act of 1925, which handed administration of these gurdwaras back to the Shiromani Gurdwara Parbandahk Committee (SGPC) – an elected body dominated by the Akali Dal party and which continues to dominate the religious and political affairs of the Sikh Panth. An important milestone for the SGPC was the publication of the *Sikh Rahit Maryada*, or the Sikh Code of Conduct, in 1953, which guaranteed greater uniformity of Sikh religious and ethical practices (Oberoi 1994).

Beliefs and practices

General

The distinctive nature of Sikhism can be traced to the thought of Guru Nanak which is embodied in his hymns that are part of the Adi Granth, amplified in the lives and works of his nine successors, and explained in the interpretations of Sikh scholars. For devout Sikhs, the most succinct articulation of Nanak's thought is encapsulated by the expression *ik oankar*, which appears at the very beginning of Nanak's *Japji Sahib* (the first and most authoritative hymn in the Adi Granth). This phrase is often translated as "One God Exists," though it is better translated as "The One Absolute Manifested Through Primal Word-Sound." According to Guru Nanak, the Absolute is non-dual (One). From the human standpoint, however, the Absolute is often perceived dualistically in terms of either/or distinctions such as *nirgun/sargun* (without qualities/with qualities; formless/ form), or in terms of the difference between God and humans. But according to Guru Nanak, the Absolute cannot be conceptualized or obtained through rituals, through mere silencing of the mind, or by satisfying one's cravings. The Absolute can only be realized through experience. To realize the One, the ego-centered individual (*manmukh*) must be grounded in a state of existence that relinquishes the individuality of the self so that when the ego, or the self, is dropped off, the person (heart/mind/soul) emerges to merge with the Absolute, or the One. In this state, the person instinctively avoids relating to the One in terms of subject and object. Such a realized individual (*gurmukh*) no longer makes a conscious distinction between I and not-I, leaving an ecstatic and purely spontaneous form of existence (*sahaj*).

In Sikh tradition, the figure of the *gurmukh* and the spontaneous freedom associated with it are seen as an intensely creative form of existence that is "oriented toward the guru" and aligned with the divine order. The transition from duality to non-duality (or the transition from *manmukh* to *gurmukh*) is made possible through *naam* (the Name). In Sikh thought, *naam* is the medium through which the ego loses itself in human communication with others and experiences non-duality. In Nanak's hymns, *naam* is not a particular word or mantra, but is both comprised and written within the vibration of the cosmos. Being the link between mystic interiority and worldly action, *naam* is experienced by the *gurmukh* through the practice of *simaran* (constant remembrance or repetition of the Name), a form of meditation in which the One simultaneously becomes the focus of an individual's awareness and their motivation to perform righteous action. However, *naam* cannot be obtained voluntarily. Its attainment depends on grace or the favorable glance of the guru which leads to change in the individual from their birth nature to the spontaneous being of the *gurmukh*.

Thus, the guru in Sikhism takes on a role that goes well beyond what the word means in Hinduism where it is limited to a teacher. In Sikhism, the term guru includes this earlier meaning and goes beyond it to refer to the same divine light manifested in the ten historic gurus. Practically it serves to indicate the authority vested in the name Nanak. Just before the death of the tenth Nanak, Guru Gobind Singh, authority was jointly vested in the Adi Granth (hence, Guru Granth Sahib) leading to the doctrine of scripture or Word as guru (*shabad-guru*) and in the collective wisdom of the initiated community, the Khalsa, giving the doctrine of panth as guru (*guru-panth*). Underpinning all of these notions is the additional notion of guru as the divine principle itself. Therefore, a guru can simultaneously be a wise teacher, scripture, community, and the divine principle that undergirds the way of the Sikh tradition.

In matters of ethics, Sikhs turn for guidance primarily to sources such as the Adi Granth (or Guru Granth Sahib), and in addition, to secondary literature such as the compositions of Bhai Gurdas, the Dasam Granth, Janamsakhis, Rahitnamas, and to a modern document, the *Sikh Rahit Maryada* (Sikh Code of Conduct). The nature of the central Sikh scripture, the Guru Granth Sahib, is ideologically fluid in the sense that it does not allow readers to easily form absolute and concrete responses to issues that they are concerned with. This is partly because of the strongly poetic nature of the text and the fact that it resists the "God–Humanity–World" schema which everyone normally associates with religion. Instead, its main focus is the transformation of the ego. Not to annihilate the ego as such, but to reach a balance between ego and ego-loss, in order to attain a certain kind of personality or state of existing-in-the-world, or *gurmukh*. To the uninitiated reader, this lack of rigid ideology and imperative (such as "you *must* do such and such") can be disconcerting. But for Sikhs it frees the individual to think outside of all constraining ideologies and to think of self almost as an artist freed to create new values, rather than simply following a set of rules. This freedom is one that takes human beings beyond simple oppositions such as good versus evil, right versus wrong, violence versus spirituality.

Despite the conceptual fluidity of the Guru Granth Sahib, the representation of the text's central teaching underwent a major revision in the early twentieth century in the hands of a neo-colonial Sikh reformist movement, the Singh Sabha. This movement was essentially a response to the proselytizing activity of Christian missionaries and to the misrepresentation of Sikh philosophy by Indologists and conservative Hindu organizations such as the Arya Samaj. The resultant modification of Sikh teaching and practice can also be seen in the way they are represented in the West, primarily in English. What we read today as "Sikh ethics," "Sikh history," or "Sikh theology" are basically responses by modern Sikhism to a colonial demand for such categories, which are not native to the Sikh tradition. Thus, in formulating ethical or religious responses to issues of health practice, one must be aware that there are differences between the approach that relies on the

Guru Granth Sahib and Sikh gurus for guidance and one that utilizes modernist ideology and methodology such the Sikh Code of Conduct (*Sikh Rahit Maryada*).

Health and disease

Disease

Disease, according to its modern conception, is an unhealthy condition, an illness or sickness of the body and mind. Such a definition presupposes that the body has a normal condition which is health and wholeness. Health, in turn, has been defined by the World Health Organization as a "state of complete physical, mental and social well-being and not merely the absence of disease or infirmity," but is more narrowly conceived by many practicing physicians as the body's physical display of vital statistics determined by medical science (Singh 2008: 32–43).

While such definitions are perfectly acceptable to Sikh philosophy, they are also far too narrow. Their narrowness results, on the one hand, from having reduced the idea of health only to what can be seen, measured, and replicated according to scientific criteria, and on the other hand, from having determined health as opposed to disease. In the teachings of the Sikh gurus, however, health and disease are ontologically connected. This is because body and mind are considered to be part of a continuum rather than opposed. Health is, therefore, imaginary if only because it is temporary. The real state of our being is "dis-ease." In this sense, disease is not episodic but chronic. Dis-ease is a condition of existing in time and the world, but without being in tune with its ebbs and flows and without realizing its transitory nature. Therefore, loss of self and the collapse of the body are normative conditions.

In Sikh scripture, disease is not always "causally" linked to a bodily mis-function, but to the way in which human beings fundamentally exist in the world – namely, the state of ego. Disease occurs when a person asserts "I am myself" and turns this enunciation of the state of being into a defensive posture resistant to the flows of nature. Thus, Guru Nanak says:

> Ego is given to man as his disease. Disease affects all creatures that arise in the world except those who remain detached. Man is born in sickness, in sickness he wanders through birth after birth. Captive to disease he finds no rest, without the Guru sickness never stops.

> (Adi Granth in Sikh.org n.d.: 1140)

In a sense this may seem to suggest that disease is incurable, or that it is not ultimately important to cure disease since any cure will be temporary. This means to perceive disease and the person who is marked with disease not as that terrifying other that must be stigmatized and isolated, but rather as something or someone who is already part of myself. Does this mean, then, that disease is simply illusory and that the pursuit of cure and of effective medicine is in vain?

On the contrary, based on the gurus' teachings on selfless giving and sacrificial care for others, Sikhs have been active in medical and philanthropic enterprises. They have also been very open to modern medical advances. The Sikh gurus, for example, vehemently rejected all manner of superstitious practices prevalent in South Asian culture, such as the belief that disease is caused by the "evil eye," black magic, or evil spirits. They also discarded the notion that disease is the result of divine punishment (Singh 2008: 35). Rather, the gurus built hospitals and sanctuaries in which they themselves worked to heal the sick, particularly those afflicted by leprosy and smallpox. Sikhs, both rich and poor, regularly donate money to build hospitals and schools in South Asia. Organ donation is a common trend amongst Sikhs and considered to be a good example of selfless giving. Such giving arises from the belief that the body is perishable and not needed in the cycle of rebirth. The real essence for Sikhs is the accumulation of memory traces that comprises one's soul. The final act of giving and helping others through organ donation is both consistent with and in the spirit of Sikh teachings.

While the medical and nursing professions are highly regarded within Sikh tradition, health practitioners should nevertheless be aware that attitudes amongst Sikhs may vary depending on the individual's level of education and social background. Also, many Sikhs are increasingly turning away from the industrial drug-based approach of modern medicine toward a more holistic view of disease. This is partly the result of a resurgence of interest in alternative modes of therapy. Reliance on homeopathic doctors is becoming increasingly common as patients become more aware of the negative side effects of modern chemical treatments. This resurgence has been aided by South Asian television programs which routinely teach yoga, Ayurvedic medicine, and other techniques to combat a large variety of ailments.

Dietary rules

Despite the fact that communal eating and the sharing of food has been and continues to be so central to the Sikh way of life, the current Sikh code of conduct (*Sikh Rahit Maryada*) has left the question of dietary rules unresolved or ambiguous at best. This is perhaps not surprising when we consider that the primary source of Sikh ethics, the Guru Granth Sahib, does not provide hard and fast rules concerning diet. Instead it offers more philosophical and pragmatic advice about avoiding or eating in moderation such foods that could potentially harm the body and mind.

Nevertheless, Sikh communities throughout the world have adopted a fairly consistent attitude toward certain kinds of food. For example, as a rule, no meat or intoxicants are served in Sikh gurdwaras (or temples), all of which have a communal kitchen attached to them. Foods prepared within the gurdwara must use wholesome natural products, primarily milk, flour from wheat or corn, and vegetables. A variety of Punjabi tea is also served in many Western gurdwaras, but this is not the norm. Sikhs initiated into certain Khalsa orders are strictly vegetarian, with one or two exceptions. The Sikh Code of Conduct does not prohibit meat eating but it does state that animals should be slaughtered as humanely as possible with a single blow. Only beef is strictly avoided as most Sikhs come from a rural background. Since the cow, buffalo, and ox were central to the livelihoods of many rural Sikhs, these animals are treated with respect and never slaughtered for consumption.

Spouse, marriage, and family

Sikhs are strongly encouraged to adopt the life of a householder. Self-realization is best achieved as a member of a family and not through withdrawal from society to become a monk or a recluse. With the exception of the child-guru Harkrishan (who died at the age of 9), all of the Sikh gurus took spouses, had children, and lived lives that combined the roles of householder, warrior, and spiritual preceptor. However, the gurus also realized that this would be the most demanding way to live. It was much easier to run away from social issues, by renouncing family ties and becoming an ascetic. Nevertheless, Guru Nanak rejected renunciation and advised his followers to:

> Remain in towns and near the main high roads, but be alert. Do not covet your neighbor's possessions. Without the Name inner poise can't be attained nor can we still our cravings. The Guru has shown me that the real life of the city, the real life of the shops, is attained by achieving inner harmony. We must be traders in truth, moderate in our eating and sleeping. This is the true yoga.
>
> (Adi Granth in Sikh.org n.d.: 939)

Echoing the strong emphasis on practicing spirituality within a worldly setting, the Sikh gurus gave women an exalted place within society. In a much-quoted verse, Guru Nanak castigates medieval Indian society for looking down on women because they menstruated or bore children. Even more vehement was the guru's condemnation of *sati*, the self-immolation of women at the funeral pyres of their husbands:

> We are born from a woman, and in a woman we grow. We're engaged to and wed a woman. We take a woman as lifelong partner, and from the woman comes family. If one woman dies we seek another. Without woman there is no social bond. So why denigrate woman when she gives birth to kings? Woman herself is born of woman, none comes into the world without her.
>
> (Adi Granth in Sikh.org n.d.: 473)

Other Sikh gurus further emphasized the status of women. Guru Amardas forbade women to veil their faces, while Guru Gobind Singh invited his spouse to become part of the ceremony for initiating Sikhs into the order of the Khalsa. In keeping with this, monogamy is therefore the preferred and predominant model. Widow remarriage is a relatively prevalent occurrence in contemporary Sikh society, although many other Sikh women choose not to remarry and remain single.

Sikhism encourages and generally follows a heteronormative model of marriage as a way to lead a wholesome life with a full expression of one's emotional, psychological, and biological impulses. However, because the joint or extended family is still the prevalent norm within North Indian society and even in the Western Sikh diaspora, marriage is not a private affair between two individuals. Rather it involves the joining of two families who become connected through the individuals. The concept of marriage in Sikhism is not based on a social contract but aims at the fusion of two souls into one. It is therefore analogous to the union of humankind with the divine, which is also the goal of Sikh spirituality. In this union humans are the lover (hence female) while the divine is the beloved (hence male). Marriage is the institution where spirituality is consummated: "They are not man and wife who have physical contact only. Only they are truly married who have one spirit in two bodies" (Adi Granth in Sikh.org n.d.: 788). Physical consummation is therefore to be considered a necessary step toward a broader goal of awakening spiritual desire and longing for detachment within the very institution which joins two individuals. Such attachment, which is to be attained while being attached to another, is likened to the "blissful state" in which the mind attains union with the beloved.

Gender and sexuality

The representation of Sikhs in the Western media – bearded and turbaned men carrying swords and cases of female infanticide – gives the impression that Sikh society is patriarchal and misogynistic. Closer scrutiny suggests, however, that the role and status of women are more diverse and influential than portrayed in the media. Women have the same access to religious teachings and practices as men, and the transmission of basic spiritual and moral precepts to the next generation usually begins with women in their role as mothers. Though rarely acknowledged, the teachings of the Sikh gurus suggest that women have an innately greater spiritual potential than men. This is partly because the central obstacle in spiritual attainment is not simply the ego but the conflation of the ego, which is thought to be a typical attribute of maleness. This attribute hinders one's ability to tap the reservoir of emotions and moods necessary for achieving a balanced state of mind. Moreover, the nature and concept of God in the teachings of the Sikh gurus is not necessarily male. Divinity has equally feminine attributes.

Historically, women have risen to the highest positions in Sikh society. The tenth guru's spouse, Mata Sundari, not only played a key role in the creation of a new spiritual-cum-military order (the Khalsa), but after the guru's death led the Sikh community in spiritual and political matters, far longer than any male Sikh guru. Other women such as Rani Jindan (the spouse of the Sikh ruler Maharajah Ranjit Singh) wielded enormous power in the Sikh kingdom prior to British rule. In recent years, Bibi Jagir Kaur was elected the *jathedar* of the Akal Takht, the highest ecclesiastical position in Sikhism. All this has been possible because there are no scriptural or theological restrictions placed on women from having access to education or social, political, or spiritual ascendancy. Factors that prevent women from public endeavors have been due to the patriarchal culture of North Indian society.

Homosexuality

According to the value system of modern Sikhism as prescribed by the Sikh Code of Conduct (1954), Sikhs are expected to live in a family environment in order to properly nurture their children. Most Sikhs interpret the family structure to be based on a heteronormative model of sexuality. Many Sikhs have interpreted this to mean that homosexuality cannot result in procreation and is therefore unnatural. However, such a judgment bears a strongly Christian and especially Catholic imprint, which believes in natural law: "what is natural is what is moral." This can be seen in recent statements by Sikh religious leaders who not only openly condemned homosexuality as unnatural but seemed to justify their stance by reference to "other major world religions."

As a result of these strictures, many Sikhs with homosexual orientation have tried to enforce upon themselves "normalization" of their sexuality by convincing themselves that what they experience is merely lust and by marrying a member of the opposite sex and producing children. Such a process of forcing homosexuals to "go underground," as it were, has led to a belief among many Sikhs that there are no homosexual Sikhs. This belief can, in turn, cause distress to those Sikhs who happen to find themselves attracted to members of the same sex.

However, a closer look at the primary source of Sikh ethics, the Guru Granth Sahib, shows that while the question of homosexuality has not been explicitly discussed, there is no justification whatsoever for castigating and banning homosexuality. Moreover, South Asian culture has been traditionally tolerant toward the question of homosexuality, seeing it as one of the manifestations of ecstatic and erotic mysticism. Trans-sexuality and gender crossing is a well-known aspect of mystical enunciation, particularly in those movements influenced by bhakti (the path of devotion) and Sufism (mystical tradition in Islam). Many liberal Sikhs have called for new ways of interpreting Sikh scripture on the question of gender and sexuality which give greater credence to the trans-gendered "standpoint" of devotional love that is central to the Sikh gurus' teachings. Recent research suggests that such new interpretations are likely to complicate the issue considerably as the Sikh gurus' writings on love and eroticism may challenge the modern understandings of sexuality.

Abortion

The Sikh scriptures, the modern Sikh Code of Conduct, and related historical sources are silent about the question of abortion. As a result, individual Sikhs and Sikh communities in Punjab and in the Western diaspora have had to work out relevant responses based on their interpretation of the teachings of the Sikh gurus or by resorting to existing Punjabi cultural norms and shared traditions.

The Sikh scriptures do address important questions about the cycle of life and death that inform one's decision on abortion. It teaches that there is no absolute beginning or end to life, but that life continues beyond death in the form of a new birth. Thus, Sikhs who take the implications of this teaching seriously tend to believe that the moment of conception represents the rebirth of a fully developed person who has lived in previous lifetimes. To terminate a birth through abortion, then, would be tantamount to refusing a soul entry into a particular body and sending it back into the cycle of births and deaths – a choice that is not for human beings to make.

However, such a view is increasingly recognized by Sikhs today as idealistic and unable to provide suitable answers to instances when the mother's physical or psychological health is threatened, when there are problems with the fetus' health, or when the mother simply wishes to abort the fetus. Taking note of the fact that the vast majority of scriptural teachings do not directly address the issue of abortion, Sikhs influenced by the modern reformist tradition tend to interpret the gurus' teachings in a more pragmatic fashion. This pragmatism itself is grounded in the gurus' recognition of the mystery of life and death:

> None is informed, my trader friend, when death will come to send them off. When death comes to send them off is known to the Lord and no one else. Your family's lamentation is false, for the dead one is no longer their kin. What you get in the end is only that on which you fastened so much love.
>
> (Adi Granth in Sikh.org n.d.: 74)

Consequently, neither modern Sikh society nor its religious authorities are concerned with laying down a rigid rule on abortion. But if there is a stricture regarding abortion which would be binding on all Sikhs, it would be that abortion should not be linked to any kind of personal gain, economic or otherwise, nor driven by selfish motives or by the five traditional vices of lust, anger, covetousness, attachment, and pride. Nonetheless, doctrinal ambiguity has had one significant negative social consequence in Sikh society – that of the continuing prevalence of female feticide (Coward and Sandhu 2000: 1167). This stems from a general bias in favor of males over females, which reflects Indian society's view of women, due to the dowry system, as economic liabilities. Elective abortion for this reason has been noted even among Sikh communities in North America. Though not an uncommon practice, this type of abortion would be considered acceptable for most Sikhs.

Contraception and reproductive technologies

For Sikhs there are a number of interlinked issues to consider with regard to contraception and reproductive technologies. How is life defined, particularly in Sikh scripture? If one could define life as such, at what point does life actually begin in the reproductive timetable? And is there a moral difference between not starting a life (contraception) and ending one (abortion)? As we have seen, although the scriptures are non-committal on this topic, there are hints that the definition of life is relatively fluid and would incorporate a continuum that includes non-sentient and sentient forms. According to the writings of the Sikh gurus, a properly moral issue can only arise when a new life becomes sentient. Even though sentience includes both unconscious and conscious states of existence, the crucial point of origin may not necessarily be the physical joining of sperm and ovum, but a later stage when the fetus becomes sentient. The difficulty of pinning this process down might explain why Sikhs are not acutely concerned about contraception except insofar as it becomes an act that results from and leads to one or more of the five vices. In addition, it is also helpful to remember that women in rural India have long used alternative techniques and traditional remedies to prevent conception and carry out abortions. Thus, contraception and abortion are not linked strongly to religious concerns as they may be in other cultures.

Given the strong emphasis in Sikhism on the family, the use of research and technology is generally considered an asset. With the Sikh Code of Conduct being generally silent on the issue of technology, Sikhs are likely to welcome new technologies such as *in vitro* fertilization. Although issues such as genetic engineering have not been routinely discussed in the community, given the non-dogmatic nature of the Guru Granth Sahib, Sikhs are unlikely to be opposed to such research given its potential to predict and eradicate cases of chronic disease such as Parkinson's disease, multiple sclerosis, Down syndrome, and various types of cancer. Nevertheless, the current prevalence of female feticide in many Sikh and Punjabi households highlights the way in which reproductive technologies, such as those that enable parents to predict the sex of the fetus, can be used for purposes of questionable ethics.

Death and dying

Death is a powerful and abiding theme in the teachings of the Sikh gurus and more broadly within South Asian spirituality. Despite saying much about the fact and phenomenon of death, the Sikh gurus also acknowledge that death is and will remain a constant mystery, an irresolvable contradiction, not the least because death is intrinsically connected to life and existence rather than being opposed to it. Death and life are often mentioned and discussed in the same verse and often in the same line. In this sense the Sikh gurus perceive death differently from modern science, which defines death as the end of life caused by stoppage of the means of sustenance to body cells. In Sikh teachings, death underlies one's existence from the very start of life. As Guru Nanak says, "we entered this world with death written as our fate" (Adi Granth in Sikh.org n.d.: 1126).

One of the key terms used for death is *kal*, which has a dual signification, connoting death as well as time. Both are philosophically and psychologically intertwined. *Kal* is often denoted as *jam kal* (Jama being the Vedic god of death). To the person who refuses to confront the true nature of time as here and now, the gurus project the intolerable face of time as one's own mortality. Through this depiction one is existentially confronted with the presence of death here and now. While ordinarily people lament the passing of time, grieving for things lost, and suffering when attachments are broken, the guru teaches that attachment and suffering result only from our habitual obstruction of the natural flow of time. By accepting time's impermanence as our own essence and seeing every attempt to control it as ultimately illusory, the individual can be released from suffering even while still living and thereby attain union with the divine. This is referred to as learning to die while still living (Adi Granth in Sikh.org n.d.: 935).

Death is therefore not only the privilege of those who live life positively. It also marks the moment of union with the divine and the passage to the next birth. As such, it is not an occasion for grief. The desires, thoughts, and actions in any particular lifetime leave their traces in the memory of an individual. These traces influence the circumstances and predispositions experienced in future lives.

This non-linear, non-attached perspective on life and death sustains the practical way in which Sikhs deal with death. Since the body is useless after death, Sikhs practice cremation. Burial at sea is also permitted. After cremation, the ashes may be buried but normally the remains are dispersed into the nearest river. The cremation ceremony is a family occasion. The body is washed and clothed by members of the family who take care to ensure that it carries the symbols of the faith (*panj kakkar*, or the five Ks). The body is then taken to a cremation ground in India, or if the funeral happens to take place outside India, to a funeral home. During the journey, the mourners will sing hymns from Sikh scripture. During the cremation itself, the evening hymn is sung and the ceremony concludes with a prayer. On returning to the home of the deceased, the mourners begin a complete reading of the Guru Granth Sahib. Once the reading is completed over a period of 48 hours, the mourners will receive *karah parshad*, a sacramental food. The sharing of this food symbolizes the continuity of life in the midst of death.

Sikhs believe that human birth is a precious gift, an opportunity with which to harness the body's potential for adoring *naam* and serving others. Life is a field upon which the self can properly experience the twin registers of *sukh* (pleasure/enjoyment/happiness) and *dukh* (pain or suffering) as thoroughly intertwined. Although one's existence may be imbued with pain, Sikh teachings emphasize that one should not reject pain by labeling it bad, but rather accept it with the same demeanor that one accepts pleasure. From such a perspective, many Sikhs argue that taking one's own life is ethically wrong because the impulse to annihilate oneself emanates primarily and paradoxically from deep-seated self-attachment, the desire to cling to one's own life as if it were one's own to begin with. Moreover, suicide far from solving anything creates more pain for those left behind.

The case of euthanasia is more complex, however. To begin with, it is necessary to differentiate between active and passive euthanasia. Whereas active euthanasia implies the intentional hastening of death by a deliberate act, passive euthanasia can refer to the intentional hastening of death through a deliberate omission or withdrawal of things that might otherwise sustain life. Furthermore, euthanasia can be carried out against the wishes of the patient or actually be requested by the patient and undertaken by a third party such as a doctor. The modern and conventional Sikh response to euthanasia is to say that the decision to kill or ascribe death to a person in pain or undergoing other forms of suffering is based on delusion. The causal root of delusion can be traced to one or another of the five vices spoken of in Sikh scripture (Singh 1983: 31). In such cases, as the argument goes, the dying person and/or the person assisting the dying person should use the process of dying as an opportunity to reflect on the nature of self-attachment and other psychological charges associated with the five vices. The idea here is that as long as there is life, there is always hope. Sikhs contemplating euthanasia are encouraged to look at the whole of life and try to make the appropriate distinctions between ending life and not artificially prolonging a terminal state. For those who contemplate assisting the death of another, the emphasis of this argument is to provide greater care and service for others who are less fortunate.

While this theory works perfectly well in the cases where the motive for hastening death is physical suffering, complications can arise when we take into account other potential motives for hastening death. There are several historically important cases of Sikhs refusing to live in order to serve a noble cause, such as individuals who hasten their own death in order to save others. Two of the Sikh gurus (Arjan and Tegh Bahadur) willingly chose to be tortured and die rather than prolong their own lives and in so doing condemn their fellow men and women to subservience and misery. Their deaths had a powerful emancipatory force on the community. There are numerous other such examples in early and modern Sikh history. Of course, such death is normally classified as martyrdom, and not as euthanasia. But how distinct, philosophically and spiritually, is the concept of martyrdom from other types of death, especially when the idea of a good or proper death is so strong in Sikh scripture? Health practitioners may need to be aware, on the one hand of the psychological motivations for an individual desire to hasten death,

Table 9.1 Dos and don'ts

Dos	Don'ts
1. Be sensitive to same-gender care.	1. Do not interrupt patients during prayer.
2. Respect modesty and privacy in patient care.	2. Do not remove hair from any part of the patient's body without consulting.
3. Respect personal space by limiting physical contact.	3. Do not insist on using only hospital gowns for Sikh women.
4. Be sensitive to the religious symbols of the five Ks: uncut hair (*kesh*), a wooden comb (*kangha*), a steel bracelet (*kara*), underwear (*kachhehra*), and a ceremonial sword (*kirpan*).	4. Do not offer meat used in religious sacrificial ceremonies or Halal meat to Sikh patients.
5. Consult Sikh religious leaders/family in dealing with ethical issues.	
6. Allow family to follow tradition when preparing a dead body for the funeral.	

and on the other of the deeply spiritual and often ambivalent nature of Sikh teachings on death.

Conclusion

Sikhism preaches the message of the One True God and the path leading to oneness with God through devotion, meditation, and elimination of one's ego. Sikhs' way of living also includes living a righteous life through promoting equality, resisting discrimination, and avoiding superstition. Religion is central to the practice of health and wellness since health is not merely defined by physical functionality but alignment with the ultimate goal in life, the path to the One True God, and disease therefore is understood as a state of dis-ease due to the attachment with the ego. From this perspective, Sikhism sees medical advancement as an instrument for compassion that is in accord with Sikhs' belief in living a righteous life. Hence, within a clinical context, understanding and being intentional about religious beliefs and practices can greatly benefit Sikh patients in their recovery.

Case study #1

An 18-year-old male presented to the emergency department with a laceration near his groin. During intake, making light conversation, the nurse asked him if he followed the Sikh religion. The nurse thought she recognized the special head covering the patient wore.

After what seemed like hours, the patient was taken to a room inside the ED where another nurse, a male, performed the initial exam, which included cleaning the laceration. The nurse told the patient that Dr. Charity Nboko would be in shortly to take a closer look at the wound as it likely would require sutures.

When the nurse was about to exit the room, the patient politely requested that the male nurse perform the examination and suturing instead of the female doctor. The patient further requested that no female providers be in the room while his undergarment, including his turban (*pagri*), were removed.

Questions for reflection

1. What about the Sikh tradition might explain the patient's reservations about removing his undergarment? What is the Sikh-specific name for this undergarment and what does it symbolize?
2. Name at least two additional religious traditions where religious concerns around modesty may arise clinically.
3. How can the providers best honor this request while providing patient-centered care?

*Submitted by Garrett Potts

Case study #2

Violence perpetrated by patients toward caregivers is an increasing problem all across the US. City Memorial Hospital in Yourtown, TX recently installed metal detectors in their three main entrances: the ER, the main lobby, and the surgical suite.

The Sidhu family was celebrating their recent newborn child, a healthy baby girl. Avani was charming the entire family. Three generations of the family had come to town to be present for Avani's birth. Grandfather Suraj Sidhu was particularly happy because even though the family all now lived in Texas, they were still very invested in maintaining their Sikh faith and family traditions. Avani's father came down to the main lobby to greet his Suraj and help him up to the Mother/Baby unit for a visit.

Their excitement came to a screeching halt when the metal detector started flashing lights and beeping like the end of the world was here! The intimidating security officer in full uniform with a firearm on his belt approached Suraj with a metal detecting wand as the detector attendant asked Suraj if he had any metal items in his pockets. He and Avani's father smiled and laughed when they realized Suraj had worn his *kirpan* (ceremonial knife) as he always does. This is what had set off the metal detector.

The security guy found its location, low, on the right side of Suraj's waist near his right pants pocket. He explained to the officer that it was completely wrapped up and unreachable under all the rest of his clothes. Furthermore, it was one of the dull ones, completely unable to cut anything because it was for religious purposes. The security officer was unmoved. He told Suraj that he either took it off and left it with them or he would not be able to enter the hospital.

Questions for reflection

1. If you were the hospital administrator with oversight of security, would you make an exception for Sikhs carrying *kirpans*?
2. If Sikhs can carry kirpans into the hospital, why wouldn't Native Americans be allowed to conduct smudging ceremonies in patient rooms by making similar exceptions?
3. What is the difference, if there is one, between a Sikh carrying a ceremonial knife and an American 2nd Amendment zealot carrying a pistol through the metal detector? According to local and state laws, it is legal to carry a sidearm in public so why couldn't this person carry it in the hospital?

*Submitted by Mark F. Carr

Glossary

Adi Granth Translated as "the first" and refers to the early compilation of Sikh scriptures by the fifth Guru.

Gurdwara Gurdwara is translated as "the door/path to the Guru" and refers to the Sikh temple.

Gurmukh The idea behind *Gurmukh* is to follow the teachings of the Guru instead of giving in to one's inclination and desire.

Guru Granth Sahib This body of literature is the Sikh's holy scripture and is regarded as the final authority for all Sikhs.

Khalsa Khalsa means "pure" and refers to Sikhs who have been baptized or initiated through a special ceremony.

Sikh Rahit Maryada The code of conduct incumbent upon all Sikh faithful.

The five vices The five vices that beset human behavior are Kam (lust), *Krodh* (rage), *Lobh* (greed), *Moh* (attachment), and *Ahankar* (ego).

The five virtues The five virtues taught by Sikh Gurus are *Sat* (truth), *Daya* (compassion), *Santokh* (contentment), *Nimrata* (humility), and *Pyare* (love).

Bibliography

Coward, H., and Sandhu, T. (2000) "Bioethics for Clinicians: Hinduism and Sikhism," *Canadian Medical Association Journal, 163*(9): 1167–1170.

Mandair, Alvind Pal-Singh (2013) *Sikhism: A Guide for the Perplexed*. London: Bloomsbury.

Oberoi, H. (1994) *The Construction of Religious Boundaries: Culture, Identity and Diversity in the Sikh Tradition*. New Delhi: Oxford University Press.

Rosentiel, T. (2012) *How Many US Sikhs?* Pew Research. www.pewresearch.org/2012/08/06/ask-the-expert-how-many-us-sikhs/

Sikh.org (n.d.) *Sri Guru Grand Sahib (Adi Granth)*. (English Translation). www.sikhs.org/english/eg_index.htm

Singh, A. (1983) *Ethics of Sikhism*. Patiala: Punjabi University Press.

Singh, K. (2008) "The Sikh Spiritual Model of Counseling," *Spirituality and Health International, 9*: 32–43.

US Department of State (2018). Report on International Religious Freedom: India. State.gov. www.state.gov/reports/2018-report-on-international-religious-freedom/india/

10 Islam

Hamid Mavani

In the name of God, most benevolent, ever-merciful.
All praise be to God, Lord of all the worlds,
Most beneficent, ever-merciful. King of the Day of Judgment.
You alone we worship, and to You alone turn for help.
Guide us (O Lord) to the path that is straight, the path of those You have blessed,
Not of those who have earned Your anger, nor those who have gone astray.

(Qur'an, Sura 1, author's own translation)

The Prophet said, "Give food to the hungry, pay a visit to the sick and release (set free) the one in captivity (by paying his ransom)."

(Hadith in Sahih Bukhari n.d.)

Introduction

Unless you keep yourself entirely isolated from the news in the United States, you have been deluged in recent years with a plethora of articles and images of Muslims and Islam. The horrific 9/11 attack on the Twin Towers and the Pentagon, carried out by radical terrorists who referred to themselves as Muslims, was impossible to miss. Hopefully, you have Muslim friends or neighbors so you can balance what you are hearing and reading in the news with what you know by way of personal interactions. American culture is often referred to as Judeo-Christian, a designation that leaves out the third Abrahamic faith: Islam. American culture is more properly understood as Abrahamic and not simply Judeo-Christian, for Muslims and Islam have played a major role in shaping Western civilization's Judeo-Christian cultures, whether or not textbooks make note of this fact.

Please do not allow the popular media's skewed portrayal of Muslims and Islam to set the tone of your interaction with them – either personally or professionally. As you engage with Muslim patients and associates, you will find that both of you have many concerns and concepts in common.

Demographics

There are no precise and statistically sound demographic data available on Muslim Americans, primarily because the US Census Bureau and the United States Citizenship and Immigration Services prohibit asking questions about one's religious affiliation. However, there is a general agreement that the community's numerical strength, estimated at 3.5 to

DOI: 10.4324/9781003288862-10

7 million, is a growing phenomenon with membership in important segments of society. These estimates are based on various models with different assumptions (Pew Research Center 2017: 30, 49fn25).

There is a consensus that the country's three dominant groups are South and Southeast Asians (28%); Middle Easterners, North Africans, and Iranians (41%); and African American Muslims (20%), who report having converted later in their life, and converts from Hispanic (8%) and Caucasian background (Pew Research Center 2017: 119). These American Muslim communities are comprised of many racially and ethnically diverse groups, each of which has its own unique expressions and understanding of Islam. In contrast to Muslims in Europe, they have largely integrated into American society and face minimal tension in adopting its values and attitudes (Pew Research Center 2017: 50–62). Muslims are proud to be both Muslim and American (89%) and find no tension in this composite identity.

The Pew Research Center's July 2017 study estimated that this country's total Muslim population is 3.45 million, with a very young average age (under 40) constituting 60% of American Muslims, compared with 38% of the US adult population. On the other end of the spectrum, only 14% of American Muslims are 55 and over, compared with 36% of the US adult population (Pew Research Center 2017: 23). Fifty-eight percent have migrated from about 75 countries (with South Asia representing 20% of them), and 42% were born in the United States (Pew Research Center 2018). About 80% of them are Sunnis, Islam's dominant branch, and 15–20% Shi'a (Pew Research Center 2009: 41). But regardless of their numbers, Islam is an important feature of the American religious milieu and is the fastest-growing religion in the United States.

America's Muslim community comprises a mosaic of diverse ethnic and cultural groups that have embraced a variety of worldviews depending on how they read Islam's two foundational sources: the *Qur'an* and the Sunnah/Hadith. Sunnis regard the latter source as the record of Prophet Muhammad's words and deeds, whereas Shi'a recognize both it and the words and deeds of his designated successors (known as the Twelve Infallible Imams). All Muslims agree that the *Qur'an* is the timeless and inerrant Divine Word revealed to Prophet Muhammad over a period of 23 years, suggesting that it was intimately related to the life of the society in the Hejaz (Western Province in Saudi Arabia), as it existed during the seventh century. It occupies a central place in the life and thought of practicing Muslims, is the basis of their worldview, and is the cornerstone and foundation of their society. Thus, its precepts, moral imperatives, and spiritual values form the norms for Muslims everywhere. The textual *Qur'an* is complemented by the exemplary figure of Muhammad, whose statements, actions, and tacit approvals are found in the Sunnah/Hadith. This material, which elucidates the *Qur'an*, constitutes the second major source for Islamic law. Muslim jurists employ these two sources and other methodological tools, along with devices such as analogy, rational analysis, consensus, and consideration for the public welfare, to provide rulings and guidelines on temporal and religious aspects of life. They categorize their derived rulings according to a fivefold method of classification, as follows: obligatory (*wajib*), recommended (*mandub*), permissible (*mubah*), reprehensible or discouraged (*makruh*), and prohibited (*haram*).

History

The journey of Muslims to America can be viewed in five stages: they came (1) as explorers and guides; (2) fleeing the Spanish Inquisition during the sixteenth and seventeenth centuries; (3) as a result of the Barbary Coast wars and the slave trade on West Africa's coasts; (4) during the mid- to late-1800s, primarily from Lebanon and Syria; and (5) in waves after federal legislators removed the preferential treatment accorded to European immigrants in the US Immigration and Naturalization Acts of 1952 and 1965.

A large percentage of African Americans can trace their heritage directly back to slaves who came from West Africa and the survivors of the North African wars. Among the captured were Muslims who were literate, fluent in Arabic, articulate, and determined to retain their rich ancestral heritage. Therefore, Muslims of African descent are not a new phenomenon in America. The root sources of Islam in this country, the questions of race, and the development of a distinct African American Muslim identity are the natural outgrowth of these early Muslims and their struggle for survival, freedom, equality, and faith.

In this context, Islam, considered a different and foreign religion that had produced a supposed "color-blind" community seeking to transcend ethnicity and culture, had a great appeal to those who eventually joined the Nation of Islam and the Moorish Science Temple of America. Islam provided them with a new form of self-identification and liberation from American culture and history. The Ahmadiyya movement, which most Muslims consider heretical, was the primary avenue through which African Americans learned about Islam and gained access to its religious literature in the first decades of the twentieth century. Members of this movement skilfully drew African Americans toward mainstream Sunni Islam and distanced them from the nationalistic and anti-White connotations that were assumed in their early Muslim identity. Imam Warith Deen Muhammad (1933–2008) played a pivotal role in crystallizing and consolidating this paradigm shift. Louis Farrakhan, the Nation of Islam's current leader, represents the latter, anti-White, form of Islam still practiced by a minority of African American Muslims.

The McCarran–Walter Act of 1952, which relaxed the quota system established in 1924, was a strong incentive for Muslim immigration. The 1965 liberalization of America's immigration law provided an even greater impetus. Muslims took the opportunity to flee from the oppressive regimes found in Syria, Lebanon, Albania, Yugoslavia, Egypt, Iran, Palestine, and elsewhere in the hopes of finding better economic and educational opportunities, greater religious freedom, and family reunions. More recently, due to political upheavals and wars, many Muslims are coming from Somalia, Sudan, Afghanistan, Iraq, the former Yugoslavia, and the Persian Gulf. Based on surveys conducted by Ihsan Bagby, in 2020 there were 2,769 mosques, a 31% increase from 2010 (Bagby 2020). Islam is now perhaps America's third largest religion. Its followers are concentrated in the suburbs of such major cities as New York, Chicago, Detroit, Dearborn (Michigan), Houston, Los Angeles, San Francisco, Cedar Rapids (Iowa), and in the states of Florida, Texas, Arizona, and California (Carroll 2000: 103).

In the early phase of its development, the Muslim community focused on acquiring facilities in which they could pray and commemorate significant religious events, such as Ramadan and Eid al-Fitr, the festival that marks Ramadan's conclusion. Subsequently, they sought to inculcate Islamic teachings in their children, youth, and young adults and to ensure a proper knowledge base of Islam for all. The 1980s saw the establishment of full-time accredited schools that provided a daily one-hour instruction on the *Qur'an*, Islamic ethics, and the Islamic worldview. Subsequently, other agencies were established to provide services related to marital counselling, parenting, and other religious issues.

In the post-9/11 context, Muslims and Arabs saw their civil rights eroded and became targets of negative stereotypes and objects of ridicule and discrimination. Their demonization throughout popular culture, along with that of Islam, ingrained such images in countless Americans' minds. To deal with some of these issues, Muslims began to expand the scope of activities of their national, regional, and local institutions to present a united voice on issues of shared concern – the Muslim Public Affairs Council (MPAC), the Council on American-Islamic Relations (CAIR), the Muslim Students Association (MSA), the Islamic Society of North America (ISNA), the Institute on Religion and Civil Values (IRCV), and the Islamic Networks Group (ING). Muslims, both as individuals and as groups, also became active participants and promoters of interfaith dialogue, which is governed by the principles of mutual respect and mutual enrichment. This constitutes a significant paradigm shift, primarily in terms of toning down exclusivist claims of salvation and focusing on articulating points of convergence and commonalities. While Muslims have made substantial progress in this regard, the critical importance of intra-Muslim discourse has only recently come to prominence with the upsurge in sectarian violence in Iraq, Syria, Yemen, and Pakistan, which is usually framed as a Sunni–Shi'a feud. Islam's egalitarian worldview is also lacking when it comes to the relationship between immigrant–indigenous African American Muslims and gender equality, along with the dearth of interracial marriages and segregated ethnic-based Islamic centers despite America's pluralistic nature. However, post-9/11, substantial efforts are being made to bridge this immigrant–indigenous gap.

One of the American Muslim community's major challenges and concerns is its youth's alienation and disillusionment with their religious and cultural roots. Several reasons account for this, among them the imported religious leaders' lack of knowledge about their concerns and issues, unfamiliarity with American society, and inability to communicate effectively in English. In addition, many of them are asked to perform tasks for which they have not been trained, such as serving as counsellors, community activists, interfaith dialogue participants, fundraisers, and spokespersons for their communities and Muslims as a whole. American Muslims have recently set up accredited post-secondary institutions, like Bayan Islamic Graduate School and Zaytuna College, to produce indigenous Muslim scholars who are conversant with the academic study of religion and the seminary curriculum, and who understand the concerns and challenges posed by modernity.

A Pew survey indicated that overall, Muslims have a positive attitude toward the American public and society and believe that they can actualize their potential with equity and fairness. Many Muslim Americans (69%) consider working for justice and equality and environmental ethics (62%) integral parts of Muslim identity (Pew Research Center 2017: 63).

Beliefs and practices

General

The word "Muslim" perhaps reflects Islam's single most important belief: one who voluntarily and knowingly submits to God. Given the Abrahamic belief that God created all humans, Islam states that all humans are born "muslim." Upon reaching maturity and realizing one's dependence upon God, one then submits to His divinity and becomes

"Muslim" by stating: "There is no deity except God, and Muhammad is the messenger of God." In sum, this profession of the faith mandates the total rejection of polytheism, atheism, agnosticism, and any belief system that in some way denies strict monotheism.

Belief in Muhammad and his role as a messenger of God is also essential. Muhammad is seen as the final link in a long chain of male prophets sent by God to reveal the Truth to humanity, as one of the great prophets who brought forth significant religions and/or reform of religions, such as Noah, Abraham, Moses, and Jesus. All of these prophets are to be honored and believed, have their messages respected, and function as role models for humanity, as Muhammad himself did. What sets Muhammad and God's revelation through him apart is that he emerged within the people and cultures of the Arabian Peninsula.

In addition to freeing his people from their ancestral polytheism, Muhammad's message also urged them to accept the trust God had given them: being stewards of His creation. God willed that they model the just life and uphold His will for this world. Social justice was essential to Muhammad's early message, for he and his followers were tasked with ending the socially acceptable tribal practices of female infanticide, tribalism, and slavery. In addition, despite Islam's rapid expansion, non-Muslims were *not* to be compelled to embrace it: "There is no compulsion in religion: true guidance has become distinct from error" (*Qur'an* 2004: 2:256). A person's free choice to submit to God was celebrated, and people who valued and practiced other religions were free to continue doing so in return for paying the *jizya* tax.

The growing faith's authority settled upon two primary sources: the *Qur'an* and Muhammad's life – his personal life, practices, characteristics, and teachings. Over time, his "sayings" also became authoritative. Codified into volumes and traced back via a chain of trustworthy reporters based on personal connections, the last one of whom was agreed upon to have heard Muhammad actually say it. His words acquired a significant influence in the subsequent religious leaders' thinking and rulings. Unfortunately, these reports were gathered almost two centuries after his death and thus many experts believe they contain some fabrications and false claims.

The daily lives of Muslims also took on particular patterns as the religion developed. These orthodox practices, known as the Five Pillars of Islam, are the following: (1) the verbal testimony of one's belief in God and the Prophet (the *shahada*); (2) performing the five obligatory daily prayers (*salat*) while facing Mecca; (3) giving of alms to the less fortunate (*zakat*); (4) fasting the month of Ramadan from dawn to dusk (*sawm*); and (5) making the pilgrimage (*hajj*) to Mecca, if physically and financially able to do so. Of course, dispensations and accommodations are granted to those who genuinely cannot manage certain physical or financial aspects of these pillars.

These general beliefs explain the foundation and background of the Muslims' faith. Built upon these founding notions, Islam's leaders and adherents have established a large body of practices, both formal and informal, as well as religious and cultural, upon which they rely for day-to-day living.

Health and disease

Islam's attitude toward sexual morality differs significantly from that of other Abrahamic religions, as seen in its stand on marriage, procreation, the use of reproductive technologies, birth control, and abortion. The *Qur'an* and the prophetic literature present marriage as a divinely blessed and highly encouraged institution. The primordial disposition for mutual physical attraction between men and women is natural and must be cultivated in such a way that it leads to a healthy marriage permeated with love and mercy: "One of His signs is that He created spouses from among yourselves for you to live with in tranquillity: He ordained love and kindness between you. In this truly are signs for those who reflect" (*Qur'an* 2004: 30:21). Detaching oneself from society and celibacy are denounced as reprehensible practices to be avoided under normal circumstances. Prophet Muhammad is reported to have said: "Marriage is my tradition; whosoever dissociates from my tradition does not belong to me" (Ibn Majah 1994: "Kitab al-Nikah," Book 9, Hadith 1846) and "Marry among yourselves and multiply, for I shall make a display of you before other nations on the Day of Judgment" (Sarakhsi 1985 4:193). Although procreation is one of the primary reasons for marriage, it is not the sole reason. Others are sexual gratification and companionship, both of which have a positive connotation. However, an infertile woman is generally viewed as deficient and thus has a lower social stature. Accordingly, reproductive technologies to cure infertility are welcomed, provided they do not violate the other legal, moral, and ethical rulings formulated by Muslim jurists (e.g., using a donor's sperm and/or egg, surrogacy, viewing the opposite gender's private parts, and using the frozen embryos if one or both of the former spouses are dead or divorced [Mavani 1996: 51–52]).

Sunni jurists have issued a range of opinions on surrogacy if a wife in a polygamous relationship lacks a uterus and thus cannot bring the pregnancy to term. Opinions on whether an embryo transfer would be permissible in this particular case range from "Yes" to "Absolutely not." Likewise, Shi'i jurists offer diverse opinions. For instance, Ayatullah Sayyid Ali Sistani of Najaf, Iraq, permits the use of surrogacy provided that the artificial fertilization comprises the ovum and the sperm from a legally married couple – be it permanent or temporary (Shi'i law permits very specific types of contractual marriages). As both the mother who provided the ovum and the surrogate mother would have a claim on the child, he suggests, based on obligatory precaution, that neither of them should be excluded from this claim. Ayatullah Khamene'i of Iran goes even further by allowing married couples to donate embryos to other legally married couples who are unable to have children due to infertility, provided that the latter obtain permission from the family court (Atighetchi 2007: 150).

Coitus interruptus ('*azl*) was practiced in Mecca during the time of Prophet Muhammad, and there is no evidence that he ever prohibited it. On the contrary, there is sufficient evidence to argue that he viewed procreation as being exclusively in the Omnipotent God's hands, meaning that no human intervention could prevent it. Extrapolating from this case, jurists allow contraceptive devices, provided that they do not harm the women. However, most consider it reprehensible if there is no valid justification, such as economic hardship or time constraints, that would prevent the parents from raising the child properly. One exception is Ibn Hazm (994–1064), who viewed coitus interruptus as a form of camouflaged infanticide. Although jurists have reached consensus on using temporary forms of contraception, they prohibit permanent contraception measures, such as vasectomy and tubal ligation, that have only a negligible chance of being reversed. Tubal ligation is prohibited for healthy spouses who carry no serious hereditary diseases that can be transmitted to the fetus.

In Sunni Islam, abortion is closely tied to defining exactly when the soul enters the developing fetus. The Qur'anic story of creation is explicit: The fetus attains personhood upon the infusion of the divine breath into his/her body (ensoulment) and, as a result, the angels are told: "When I have shaped him and breathed My Spirit into him, kneel down before him" (*Qur'an* 2004: 38:72). The statements ascribed to the Prophet provide conflicting data on the precise time of ensoulment. The most common one is on the 40th day. Jurists are divided on the legality of aborting a fetus, if it presents no risk to the mother, that is less than 120 days old. Their rulings range from permission and discouragement, with a valid reason such as economic hardship or a genetically deformed embryo, to outright prohibition. A general Sunni trend is to categorically prohibit abortion 40 days after conception, except in such serious exigencies as saving the mother's life. Although one can find diverse opinions on abortion prior to the fetus' ensoulment, there is almost unanimity on the absolute prohibition of abortion after its ensoulment, except if continuing the pregnancy would kill the mother or cause her serious mental and/or physical harm (Sachedina 2009: 131–133).

Among the four Sunni schools of law, the Hanafis are most tolerant of abortion done before the fetus' ensoulment. They view it as reprehensible and abominable, but still allow it with or without a valid reason. The Malikis' position is very similar to that of the Twelver Shi'is – abortion is allowed *only* to save the mother's life. The Shafi'is allow abortion within the first 40 days, although it is considered *makruh* (strongly discouraged and detestable). The Hanbalis' position has varied from prohibition after conception to permission to abort, although it is morally reprehensible, the zygote during the first 40 days. Shi'a jurists prohibit abortion absolutely, unless it is necessary to save the mother's life.

The *Qur'an* speaks of the seven stages of embryonic development:

> We created man from an essence of clay, then We placed him as a drop of fluid in a safe place, then We developed that drop into a clinging form, and We developed that form into a lump of flesh, and We developed that lump into bones, and We clothed those bones with flesh, and later we developed him into other forms – glory be to God, the best of creators! Then you will die and then, on the Day of Resurrection, you will be raised again.
>
> (*Qur'an* 2004: 23:12–16)

Regardless of the specific issue at hand, one must keep in mind the importance of the care provider–patient relationship in Islamic thought. Both Sunni and Shi'a Islam encourage a same-sex provider–patient relationship. The concern here is to protect the virtue of both parties during routine care procedures. If this ruling is suspended due to an emergency, a family member and/or additional care providers *must* be present to prevent any possible lapse of virtue.

Death and dying

Beliefs

Free will and predestination have been discussed extensively right from the first days of Islam. This theological discussion was not strictly academic in nature; rather, it was organically related to the political legitimacy of the ruling Umayyad dynasty (661 to 750). Most of its caliphs were of low character and Muslim in name only. As a result, the community sought to evaluate the legality of their status and whether the *Qur'an* and prophetic paradigm would permit rebellion against them. The Umayyads, seeking to justify their rule, propounded the theory of divine determinism – God had bestowed leadership upon them and thus had decreed all their actions. Any attempt to overthrow them, therefore, would be a sin and a challenge to His omnipotence and comprehensive authority. This discussion took place when the dominant view was fatalism accompanied by a pessimistic notion of time as an inexorable force that will bring everything to an abrupt end. In other words, human beings have no agency in matters of death and destruction, fortune and misfortune – a worldview that the *Qur'an* specifically mocks:

> They say, "There is only our life in this world: we die, we live, nothing but Time destroys us." They have no knowledge of this; they only follow guesswork: their only argument, when Our clear revelations are recited to them, is to say, "Bring back our forefathers if what you say is true." [Prophet], say, "It is God who gives you life, then causes you to die, and then He gathers you all to the Day of Resurrection of which there is no doubt, though most people do not comprehend."
>
> (*Qur'an* 2004: 45:24–26)

Refuting such pessimism – no free will, personal accountability, and afterlife – the *Qur'an* proclaims one's earthly life a testing ground and a bridge that can lead one to a life of eternal bliss and joy in the hereafter. The only requirement is that he/she abide by the divine prescriptions. God elevated humanity as a whole by appointing both men and women as His deputies (*khalifa*; *Qur'an* 2004: 2:30) on Earth to actualize divine purpose: enabling humans to move toward perfection by establishing a just social, moral, ethical, and spiritual order so that they will achieve felicity and prosperity in this life and the afterlife. Accordingly, physical death does not mean that humans cease to exist, for their virtuous deeds will bear fruits in the afterlife. In one tradition, Prophet Muhammad is reported to have said: "This life is a farm to cultivate for the hereafter" (Rayshari 2001: 2:895).

The *Qur'an* states that humans are composed of two contradictory elements: divine spirit (*Qur'an* 2004: 32:7) and mud or clay (ibid.: 3:59 and 7:12). The divine breath and the primordial nature (*fitra*) generate motivation toward that which is lofty and sublime. The second ingredient, mud, turns humans toward lowliness and the unbridled fulfilment of base desires. Humanity received the knowledge of good and evil via "revealed books" (the Abrahamic scriptures) brought and exemplified by the prophets' lives, their primordial nature (*fitra*) (*Qur'an* 2004: 91:8–9), and the "book of nature," which points toward the existence of God, the only one worthy of adoration, worship, and submission (ibid.: 10:6–7). Humanity's freedom of choice elevates its members' status in relation to the angels, who do not enjoy this distinction. In short, nobility is contingent upon the bestowal of free will and knowledge, as opposed to any natural and racial characteristics. God summons humans to develop a bond with Him and perform noble deeds that will ensure a blissful afterlife for them.

Islam rejects the Christian doctrine of Original Sin. In fact, one can argue that it teaches Original Purity, because every person is born with a clean conscience and a primordial disposition to abide by the universal moral and ethical values. In a prophetic tradition, Muhammad says: "Every child is born on his natural state of good conscience" (Sarakhsi 1985: v.11: 246). The *Qur'an* presents everyone as being created with an inclination toward virtue as well as being capable of going against this natural tendency by being inevitably attracted to satanic temptations and, as a result, committing sins. However, all sins can be forgiven prior to death and the loss of agency (*Qur'an* 2004: 39:53 and 4:31), including the greatest sin of all – polytheism or associationism (*shirk*) (ibid.: 4:48) – provided that the person sincerely seeks forgiveness, renounces the evil act, regenerates virtuous desires and intentions, and provides restitution to the wronged party. The *Qur'an* 7:20–22 and 20:121 identifies the first moral/ethical violation, that of Adam and Eve, as following Satan's prompting to eat from the forbidden tree. But, as distinct from the Biblical account, God forgave both of them: "Then Adam received some words from his Lord and He accepted his repentance: He is the Ever Relenting, the Most Merciful" (*Qur'an* 2004: 2:37). Thus, there is no transmission of "original error" or "sin" to their posterity, or a permanent abandonment from God.

As mentioned earlier, Islam views life on Earth as a prelude and a precursor to the eternal life in the hereafter, as well as a preparatory phase before returning back to our origin: "We belong to God, and to Him we shall return" (*Qur'an* 2004: 2:157). The *Qur'an* often underlines the inevitability of each person's death and ultimate return to God for accountability and meeting Him. The major phases of a human being's life are mentioned as follows: "How can you ignore God when you were lifeless and He gave you life, when He will cause you to die, then resurrect you to be returned to Him?" (*Qur'an* 2004: 2:28).

By breathing His divine breath into all human beings, God gave them life, dignity, and trusteeship over their bodies. This trust is not absolute however, just as a person's ownership of worldly things is not absolute. As such, issues dealing with the termination of life require the consent and the endorsement of God, the absolute Trustee and Creator of human life.

Defining the exact point when life commences and terminates is fraught with difficulties and challenges because the revelatory sources are not explicit in these matters. However, one thing is clear: God is the author of life and death. Several Qur'anic verses state that a person's lifespan and death are pre-determined, just as his/her sustenance has already been pre-recorded: "No person grows old or has his life cut short, except in accordance with a Record: all this is easy for God" (*Qur'an* 2004: 35:11) and "No soul may die except with God's permission at a predestined time" (ibid.: 3:145). Works dealing with death focus on the soul after it has separated from the body, as opposed to defining the moment of death in other than general terms.

However, Islamic legal theory contains the following basic rule: Jurists should defer to experts in the relevant field(s) to acquire an authoritative understanding of the involved definitions. So, for instance, they should rely on experts to identify the correct direction for the five daily obligatory prayers and for positioning the deceased in his/her grave toward Mecca. Likewise, they should rely upon astronomical evidence to ascertain the birth of a new crescent moon when the Moon is blocked by clouds. Accordingly, jurists must consult doctors when determining the valid criteria for death, especially since traditional understandings, based primarily on external evidence largely derived from human experience, have been rendered obsolete due to modern technology's ability to sustain some form of organ activity.

Upon the onset of death, Islamic teachings recommend the performance of certain rituals to facilitate the soul's departure from the patient's body, to safeguard it from undergoing hardship and torment, and to re-confirm the patient's covenant with the Creator by reciting the testimony of faith: "There is no god except one God, and Muhammad is the messenger of God." During this time, the Islamic rules regarding gender segregation and modesty must be observed. Family members must be informed of the patient's impending death so they can be close by to offer comfort and solace, as well as to encourage the patient to repent of his/her sins and seek God's forgiveness. Leaving the dying patient alone or to weep and wail uncontrollably is discouraged and reprehensible, for such behavior implies that he/she is fighting God's decree. In addition, Muslims customarily recite certain chapters of the *Qur'an*, such as Yasin (chapter 36) and the Confederates (chapter 33), to remind the dying of his/her covenant with God and His messenger. The Shi'a add the Twelve Infallible Imams or Guides. The dying person should be positioned such that his/her soles face the Ka'bah in Mecca. After his/her death, the corpse can be left in that state until it is taken away for the ritual washing, funeral prayers, and burial. In Sunni Islam, it can be laid at a perpendicular angle so that the Ka'bah is to the dying person's right. Muslims believe that one who has lived a life anchored in Islam's moral and ethical worldview and has benefitted humanity will be greeted by the Angel of Death with the following words: "O you, soul at peace: return to your Lord well pleased and well pleasing; Go in among My servants, and into My Garden" (*Qur'an* 2004: 89:27–30).

After the patient has died, one should close the mouth, fasten the jaw with a strip of cloth so the mouth cannot open, straighten the hands and the legs, cover the corpse with a clean sheet of cloth, and pray. The corpse must be treated with respect and dignity because, it is argued, it can still feel the pain as the soul is still connected to it. The deceased Muslim woman is still entitled to enjoy the rules of modesty as if she were still alive. The rituals associated with washing, shrouding, praying, and burying the deceased cannot be delayed. Consequently, the necessary religious requirements should be arranged as quickly as possible, normally by the person delegated by the deceased. All Muslims are responsible for providing the burial service, but this responsibility ends as soon as someone or a group fulfils it. If this obligation remains unfulfilled, then everyone is considered guilty of sinning and held religiously accountable. If the deceased is aged four months or less, the only requirements are that they be wrapped in a piece of cloth and buried.

After these rituals have been carried out, Islamic tradition states that the soul will re-enter the corpse on the first night after its burial so that he/she can be questioned by two angels – Munkar and Nakir – on their testimony of faith in God and His messenger (and, in Shi'ism, the Twelve Infallible Imams as well), the *Qur'an*, the angels, and the Day of Judgment. If successful, the grave will be expanded and made spacious and the deceased will be able to smell the breeze from paradise until the Day of Resurrection. If unsuccessful, it will become narrow and full of torment, a foretaste of the punishment awaiting him/her in the hell-fire. This period is known as *barzakh*, the barrier between death and resurrection or, as some scholars have named it, the intermediate world of imagination.

Practices

The *Qur'an* explicitly asserts that only God, the originator of life, has the right to terminate it: "[O Prophet], say, 'It is God who gives you life, then causes you to die, and then He gathers you all to the Day of Resurrection of which there is no doubt, though most people do not comprehend'" (*Qur'an* 2004: 45:26). The misguided idea that one can delay death is denounced as human arrogance: "When a person's term comes to an end, God never grants a reprieve. God is fully aware of what you do" (*Qur'an* 2004: 63:11). Such statements are not intended to promote fatalism, but to reflect God's all-comprehensive authority and knowledge, as well as His awareness of everything that each person's freedom of choice will cause him/her to do.

Islam prohibits suicide on the grounds that life is sacred and a divine trust, and that any violation of this trust is, in addition to arrogating God's role to oneself, no more than arrogance and ingratitude for His favors and bounties. Committing suicide while despondent and hopeless is condemned as being ungrateful and fighting the divine will. Thus, it falls under the category of major sins. The Prophet is reported to have said that one who commits this act will be subject to eternal punishment by being consigned to the hellfire with no chance of reprieve. The *Qur'an* admonishes people to "Spend in God's cause: do not contribute to your destruction with your own hands, but do good, for God loves those who do good" (*Qur'an* 2004: 2:195).

Life on Earth is viewed as a testing ground where humans will be afflicted with trials and tribulation in the form of loss of lives, property, and economic stability: "We shall certainly test you with fear and hunger, and loss of property, lives, and crops. But [O Prophet], give good news to those who are steadfast" (*Qur'an* 2004: 2:155). While we may not be able to understand why we or others are suffering, there is always an underlying rationale and wisdom for it, because God is neither so capricious nor unkind as to send us a pointless trial. Some prophetic traditions refer to cleansing one's sins or providing an example for the living as possible reasons. Moreover, enduring these challenges with patience and forbearance is a sign of one's strong conviction.

At the same time, using palliative care to reduce one's suffering and improve the quality of life is encouraged. In early Islamic legal literature, active forms of euthanasia or physician-assisted suicide were often equated with suicide. Little or no distinction was made between the two, and this remains the case today. Present-day scholars implicitly allow passive forms of euthanasia by interpreting it as a sign of one's resignation to the divine will. This position can be further buttressed by arguing that delaying an inevitable death via invasive procedures is contrary to the patient's interest to die with dignity when his/her life no longer has any merit, whether to self or to society and, moreover, uses up valuable resources that could be channeled elsewhere.

This ruling can also be applied in the case of brain-dead patients or situations where there is no hope of survival. Such passive forms of euthanasia are withholding certain treatments that would only delay one's imminent death, not connecting the patient to a lifesaving apparatus, or administering drugs that alleviate pain but may accelerate the patient's death. Twelver Shi'i jurists have not reached unanimity on the legality of withdrawing the life-support apparatus once it has been connected to the patient and activated. The breakneck pace of advances in medical technology are forcing the jurists to formulate new definitions of death. It goes without saying that each decision made by physicians requires the consent of the patient and the immediate family, or the person designated to make decisions on his/her behalf.

Islam states that the corpse is to be treated with respect, dignity, and honor even after the soul has left it. As such, performing an autopsy or a post-mortem investigation, donating one's organs, and using bodily organs to help doctors find cures for other ailments have traditionally been prohibited in order to preserve the body's integrity, appearance, and dignity. However, the principle of public welfare (*maslaha*), in which the benefits outweigh the demerits, is causing such rulings to be re-evaluated. In the past,

Table 10.1 Dos and don'ts

Dos	Don'ts
1. Ask if the patient would like privacy to pray.	1. Do not feed the patient anything that contains pork or alcohol or any of their by-products.
2. Ask if the patient would prefer male or female providers.	2. Do not assume that religious traditions are unimportant.
3. Ask if the patient would like help contacting the local imam (Sunni or Shi'a).	3. Do not assume that performing the obligatory prayers is irrelevant while in the hospital.
4. Inform the dietician of food consumption rules, like meat (*zabiha*) that is slaughtered in the Islamic manner.	4. Do not send an opposite-sex caregiver into the patient's room alone.
5. Make sure the family is included in decision-making discussions.	

jurists were mindful of the sanctity of a Muslim's corpse and thus would advise that their bodies be spared if there are volunteers among the unbelievers who would fulfil the need. But there is clearly an ethical problem here, given the Islamic concept of universal human dignity regardless of religion: "We have honoured the children of Adam [and Eve] and carried them by land and sea" (*Qur'an* 2004: 17:71). Thus, some jurists have argued that since all life and bodies are equally precious and sacred, no distinction should be made between Muslims and non-Muslims. Autopsy would be permitted if the law of the land mandates it or the merits of doing so outweigh the demerits. Cremation, on the other hand, is strictly prohibited and not open for discussion or analysis.

Conclusion

Given the conjoined seminal history of the three Abrahamic faiths, it is not surprising that so much of what we have learned in this chapter on Islam is similar to what we find in Judaism, and Christianity. Aside from the variety of positions we see within Islam, the general frame of reference to God and His revealed word through Prophet Muhammad remains central. Healthcare professionals who respect the views of practicing or cultural Muslims will be a step ahead when it comes to providing them with the appropriate medical care.

Case study #1

A married couple were settling into the hospital's postpartum unit after the birth of their first child. The husband asked that no males be allowed to enter their room. The nurse assured the father that a sign would be placed on the door stating that no male was to enter and to check at the nurses' station with any questions.

A male lab tech, assigned to draw postpartum labs on the mother, read the sign on the door and angrily approached the nurses' station for an explanation. The nurse explained that the husband had requested that no males be allowed in the room. "This is stupid, I need to do my job and that includes drawing labs," the tech asserted. The nurse responded, "You cannot enter the room. A female lab tech will be the only person allowed to enter the room to draw labs." Again, the tech urged, "I have a job to do, and

I don't know that there are any female techs available." The nurse countered, "I find it hard to believe that there are not any female techs available. Regardless, you will not enter the room." The male tech left muttering under his breath that this was stupid.

Questions for reflection

1. Was the lab tech guilty of overt prejudice or just ignorance? If ignorance, who is responsible for his education? If prejudice, what should be the consequences?
2. What situations or emergencies might override the father's request that males not be allowed to enter the room?
3. Must honoring a request to exclude male caregivers be based on recognized religious grounds, e.g. Muslim, Orthodox Jew, etc., or would personal convictions be sufficient? Should the mother's explicit consent be required before acceding to the father's request?
4. The demand for same gender care has been extended to physicians in the delivery room and even to radiologists examining X-rays. Where should the limits be drawn, if at all?

*Submitted by Barbara Cheuvront

Case study #2

Aabira was a 59-year-old female from Libya visiting her adult daughters in Florida. While visiting she fractured her left proximal tibia, after tripping over a curb. Without insurance and unable to afford physical therapy, she was excited to discover the pro bono clinic where I volunteered as a physical therapist. We spent two months aggressively regaining the bend in her knee and strength throughout her left leg.

One day I took measurements of the bend in her knee as well as her leg strength. She had increased the bend of her knee from 85 degrees to 120 degrees. She had also made significant strength gains. Together, these improvements would help her walk up to her fifth-floor apartment in Tripoli. Yet she still didn't seem satisfied. So, I asked if something was bothering her.

"I am very happy with the progress I have made," she replied. "But I still won't be able to bend my knee enough to get into a prayer position." I knew that she was Muslim. She wore a hijab to each of her therapy sessions. I gained permission to touch her and appropriately drape her with a sheet when I had to expose portions of her leg. Yet I had nearly missed an important element of physical therapy care. I had failed to fully consider how much her religion would impact aspects of her recovery and the knee motion goals she had set for herself.

Questions for reflection

1. According to Islamic teaching, what are the benefits, present and future, of faithfully following the prescribed prayer regimen, including the bodily positions? In Islam there are repeated references in the texts that religion should be one of ease and felicity without imposing an onerous burden. This is precisely why God has provided *rukhsah* (exemptions) for such cases. Could Aabira simply talk to her Imam and gain an exemption from normal prayer posture?

2. To return to normal prayer position, Aabira would need approximately a 140-degree knee bend. Why might she be so determined to return to her normal prayer routine?
3. Sunni Muslims are called to prayer five times a day at designated times, reciting a specific prayer with each change of body position. Orthodox Jews and some Christians pray three times daily, particularly at mealtime. What would be the point of praying before eating?

*Submitted by Jeff Emde

Glossary

Hajj The pilgrimage to Mecca that each Muslim is required to undertake at least once in her/his life, if able to do so.

Haram A forbidden act. Islamic jurists classify all human actions in five groups: *wajib* (obligatory), *mandub* (recommended), *mubah* (permissible), *makruh* (reprehensible or discouraged), and *haram*.

Hijab Modest attire that conceals a woman's beauty and bodily shape. It generally includes everything but the face, hands, and feet.

Imam A title of respect used for a Muslim community's religious leader. Parallel terms in Judaism and Christianity would be rabbi and pastor or priest, respectively.

Ka'bah The cubic structure constructed by Abraham and his son Ishmael toward which all Muslims face during prayer and which the pilgrims circumambulate together during the hajj.

Qur'an Islam's holy scripture, which was revealed to Muhammad in Mecca and Medina over the course of 23 years.

Ramadan The annual month of religious and personal devotion marked by fasting from sunrise to sunset. If they are able to do so, Muslims must abstain from food and water during the day time and, after sunset, get together with their families and friends to enjoy a delightful meal together.

Sunnah/Hadith A record of Prophet Muhammad's words, deeds, and tacit approvals. For the Shi'a, this also includes the words and deeds of his designated successors (the Twelve Infallible Imams). This body of literature constitutes the second major source of authority for Islamic law.

Zabiha The meat of an animal slaughtered in accord with Islamic dictates.

Bibliography

Atighetchi, D. (2007) *Islamic Bioethics: Problems and Perspectives*. New York: Springer.

Bagby, I. (2020) "The American Mosque: Growing and Evolving. Report 1 of the US Mosque Survey 2020: Basic Characteristics of the American Mosque," *The Institute for Social Policy and Understanding*. www.ispu.org/wp-content/uploads/2021/07/ISPU_American-Mosque-Report-1.pdf?x46312%2F

Carroll, B. (2000) "Islam in America," in *The Routledge Historical Atlas of Religion in America*. New York: Routledge.

Ibn Majah, Muhammad b. Yazid. (1994) Sunan Ibn Majah, "Kitab al-Nikah," Book 9, Hadith 1846, Beirut: Dar al-Fikr.

Mavani, H. (Trans.) (1996) "Ayatullah Sayyid Ali Sistani," in *Contemporary Legal Rulings in Shi'i Law* (pp. 51–52). Montreal: OAIK Publications, questions 137a and b.

Pew Research Center (2009) "Mapping the Global Muslim Population" www.pewresearch.org/religion/wp-content/uploads/sites/7/2009/10/Muslimpopulation-1.pdf

Pew Research Center (2017) "U.S. Muslims Concerned About Their Place in Society, but Continue to Believe in the American Dream" www.pewresearch.org/religion/wp-content/uploads/sites/7/2017/07/U.S.-MUSLIMS-FULL-REPORT-with-population-update-v2.pdf

Pew Research Center (2018) "Muslims in America: Immigrants and Those Born in U.S. See Life Differently in Many Ways" www.pewresearch.org/religion/2018/04/14/muslims-in-america-immigrants-and-those-born-in-u-s-see-life-differently-in-many-ways/

Qur'an: A New Translation (2004). (MAS. Abdel Haleem, Trans.). Oxford: Oxford University Press.

Rayshari, M. (2001) *Mizan al-Hikmah*. Qum: Dar al-Hadith.

Sachedina, A. (2009) *Islamic Biomedical Ethics: Principles and Application*. Oxford: Oxford University Press.

Sahih Bukhari (n.d.) (MM. Khan, Trans.). www.iium.edu.my/deed/hadith/bukhari/065_sbt.html

Sarakhsi, Shams al-Din (1985) *al-Mabsut*. Beirut: Dar al-Ma'rifah.

11 Judaism

Douglas Kohn

Hear O Israel, Adonai is our God, Adonai is one.

(Torah Deuteronomy 6:4)[1]

I call heaven and earth to witness before you this day, that I have set before you life and death, the blessing and the curse; therefore choose life that you may live.

(Torah Deuteronomy 30:19)

Introduction

Judaism, the oldest monotheistic religious system and the first textually based religion in the Western world, has a fundamental identification and concern with life, health, and healing. At the crowning climax of the Hebrew Bible's opening chapter (Torah Genesis 1:26–28), God formed humankind (*Adam*) in the Divine Image and charged the nascent humanity to procreate and to bear stewardship over the newly created earth. Thereafter, in the succeeding chapter which elucidates the initial creation mythology, one reads that God "breathed life into the man's nostrils" (Torah Genesis 2:7), reflecting the Deity's intimacy with humanity and fundamental ethic of concern for the life and well-being of the human being, and by extension, the human enterprise. Yet, human life, by definition, is fragile and vulnerable, and invariably the living being requires care, mediation, and support. The text of Leviticus 19:16, "Do not stand idly by the blood of your neighbor," is interpreted to compel tending and healing of the ill or injured person.

Later, in the rabbinic teachings of the Talmud (the fifth century CE code of Jewish law), the creation of Adam again is invoked to promote the primary Jewish principle of the value of life:

Therefore only a single human being was created in the world, to teach that if any person causes a single soul to perish, Scripture regards him as if he has destroyed an entire world; and if any person saves a single soul, Scripture regards him as if he had saved an entire world.

(Babylonian Talmud [BT] *Sanhedrin* 37a)

This central concept of reverence for life finds further emphasis in the liturgy for the Jewish High Holy Days of *Rosh Hashanah* (the Jewish New Year) and *Yom Kippur* (the Day of Atonement), which reads, "In the book of life … may we and all Your people …

DOI: 10.4324/9781003288862-11

be inscribed for a good and peaceful life" (Greenberg & Levine 1978: 181). One reads in the Midrash to the Hebrew Bible (a homiletic explication of the biblical text) the model of God visiting and comforting Abraham when the patriarch was healing from his circumcision (Torah Genesis 17:26–18:1, BT *Sotah* 14a), demonstrating that the process of healing is a relational, cooperative endeavor, including possibly the presence of the Holy One, but surely, human contact. Lastly, in the final book of the Torah (also known as the Pentateuch or the Five Books of Moses) is found perhaps the most commanding verse authorizing a medical ethic and the religious charge to pursue healing and life: "I call heaven and earth to witness before you this day, that I have set before you life and death, the blessing and the curse; therefore choose life that you may live" (Torah Deuteronomy 30:19). These textual references represent but a fraction of Jewish sacred scripture which serves as the foundation for a Jewish ethos of health and healing, yet each captures the common thrust: that life is cherished, and that the *mitzvah* (Divinely commanded obligation) to heal is a principal cornerstone of Jewish behavior and understanding.

One might note the large number of Jews engaged in the healing professions – as physicians, researchers, instructors, and therapists – both presently and historically, to realize the powerful influence which this ethic holds on the Jewish community. Furthermore, the Talmud teaches that it is forbidden to live in a community which lacks a physician, further compelling Jews to engage in the healing arts (BT *Sanhedrin* 17a). As much as Judaism commands the obligation to heal, it concomitantly commands the Jew to seek healing (Bleich 1981: 1–9).

Yet, Jews and Judaism are not monolithic. There is a great variety and breadth to the Jewish world and its community, with sub-streams of Jewry today spanning from the Orthodox and ultra-Orthodox sects at one extreme to Progressive and even secular Jewish streams at the opposite pole. Primarily, adherents within these Jewish sub-groups are distinguished in their respective practice and relationship to *halacha* (Jewish law), and less so in core ethics or beliefs. Some of these differences will be evident in postures toward health and medical circumstances. For the purposes of this chapter, a normative understanding and common practice are described, while noting important variations or minority examples.

Demographics

In September 2022, the Jewish Agency for Israel estimated that the worldwide Jewish population numbered approximately 15.3 million persons, although some estimates may vary due to some uncertainty in measurements and definitions. Of this population, approximately seven million Jews live in the State of Israel, and another six million live in the United States (Jewish Agency for Israel 2022). It is estimated that there are about 150,000 Jews in Russia, 446,000 in France, 399,500 in Canada, and 292,000 in the United Kingdom (DellaPergola 2021).

Metropolitan areas with significant Jewish communities include Tel Aviv (3.9 million), New York City (2.1 million), Jerusalem (993,000), Haifa (710,000), Los Angeles (622,000), Miami (535,000), Paris (338,000), Philadelphia (420,000), Buenos Aires (230,000), and London (230,000) (Jewish Virtual Library 2022).

Worldwide, two major branches represent the Jewish community of faith, the Orthodox and the Progressive, with significant sub-divisions in each branch. In the United States, the Progressive Jewish community is primarily comprised of the Reform

Movement and the Conservative Movement, with Jews of the Reconstructionist and Renewal movements representing a small fraction of Progressive Jews. The Pew Research Center (2020) "Jewish Americans in 2020" study revealed that 37 percent of America's Jews identify as Reform (2,200,000), 17 percent identify as Conservative (1,000,000), 9 percent as Orthodox (540,000), one third declare "no affiliation," and the remainder as "just Jewish." In Israel and Europe, there is only one progressive movement, commonly called "Progressive Judaism." In Israel, it is estimated that 10 percent of Jews are ultra-Orthodox, 10 percent are Progressive, and the remainder are "just Jewish," which includes a mix of Orthodox and secular Jews. In Europe, a similar ratio is found, with a smaller fraction each of Orthodox and Progressive, and the majority in the middle. Worldwide, Orthodoxy is not monolithic, either. At its extreme, small numbers of Jews are *Haredi* or *Chasidic* Jews, who adhere to a very strict, medieval interpretation of Jewish law, while the bulk are "Modern Orthodox," who fully function in modern society while maintaining Jewish ritual.

The fastest growing stream in the United States is the Reform Movement, which has been moving in its practice and philosophy nearer to the Conservative Movement, such that in many communities there is little difference between the two major movements. In America, Modern Orthodoxy is losing members, while the ultra-Orthodox is growing due to its much greater birth rate. These trends also hold in Israel, though its Progressive Movement is growing more slowly.

History

Jewish history dates to the biblical period, or the early second millennium BCE. The patriarch, Abraham (*c.*1750 BCE), is credited with being the first Jew, and from him Jewry initially grew as a familial clan of adherents to the One God, known by the Hebrew tetragrammaton (the four-letter name of God in Hebrew language), YHWH, pronounced "*Adonai*" in Hebrew, the religious language of Judaism. An initial covenant was established, linking for perpetuity this people, God, and the land of Israel. Jewish patriarchal history is detailed in the biblical book of Genesis. After a period of Egyptian enslavement, the Jews were liberated by God through the hand of Moses, known as the lawgiver (*c.*1225 BCE), and they began a journey to return to their homeland. Essential to the journey was the revelation and renewed covenant at Sinai, at which Jewish tradition credits God with giving the Torah, containing 613 commandments.

Later biblical history includes the conquest of Canaan by Joshua, Moses' successor, and the period of kings who secured and enlarged the Jewish territory, later called Judea and Samaria. King David (*c.*1000 BCE) is the most celebrated of Israel's rulers. Concurrent with the period of the monarchies was the period of the prophets, the ethical teachers who tempered the rule of the kings and spoke as intermediaries for God. Isaiah, Jeremiah, Micah, and Ezekiel are the most heralded prophets. In the sixth century BCE, the Babylonians invaded Judea and destroyed the great temple in Jerusalem, the physical and emotional center of the Jewish faith. The Babylonians returned to their homeland with the Jews in tow as prisoners. The Jewish people refer to this as the Exile, which continued until the Jews returned later that century and built the Second Temple. Jewry endured Persian and then Greek rule until the end of the second century BCE, and then revolted against the Hellenized Assyrians in the uprising which would produce the festival of Chanukah.

The Rabbinic Period commenced with the Roman Period (*c*.63 BCE–500 CE), and the Roman destruction of the Second Temple. Central to the Rabbinic Period was the discourse of the rabbis, who generated a portable, textually based religion which superseded the site-based ritualistic traditions of the Temples. The rabbis canonized the Bible, prepared the Jewish prayer book, set the festival and life cycle sequences, and wrote two codes of Jewish law, the Mishnah (redacted *c*.200 CE) and the Talmud (redacted *c*.500 CE). Essentially, the rabbis created Judaism as it is understood today. Also, with the rabbinic period came the Diaspora, or the dispersion, as Jews spread to every corner of the Roman Empire, then to all over the globe until the modern period.

For the next 1,000 years, Jews remained a minority culture under the Muslim hegemony in the Mediterranean region and the Near East, and in Christian Europe from Iberia and North Africa to Persia and India, and throughout Europe. Jews learned to live under both cultural norms. As a literate minority in the societies where they lived, Jews often served as bureaucrats, diplomats, accountants, lawyers, and physicians in both Christendom and the Muslim worlds, although Jewry was relegated to secondary status in both societies. For Jews, the height of this period was the Golden Age of Spain (*c*.900–1200 CE), during which Jews were found in the royal courts, and were the doctors and poets of the Spanish kingdoms. In 1492, King Ferdinand and Queen Isabella expelled the Jews from Spain, ending one of the greatest periods of Jewish history. The Jews of Spain, called Sephardic Jews, then emigrated and joined Jewish communities in the Mediterranean basin, and central and Eastern Europe (this later group being referred to as Ashkenazic, or German Jews).

With the modern world, Jews eventually were "liberated" and granted citizenship in the newly formed nation-states of Europe and America. In the nineteenth century, the largest population of Jews was the Ashkenazim of Eastern Europe, living in Poland and Russia's Pale of Settlement (a region in Russia where Jews settled and later were persecuted). As well, there were sizable communities in Germany and Western Europe. Due to periodic pogroms (state-sanctioned violence against Jews in the nineteenth and early twentieth centuries), many Jews immigrated to America. The tragedy of the Holocaust (1938–1945, *Sho'a*, in Hebrew), during which the Nazis murdered six million Jews, resulted in nearly every European Jewish community being decimated and nearly every Jewish family suffering loss. Following the liberation of the death camps in Europe, American Jewry would be the world's largest Jewish community. In 1948, the State of Israel was established, and Israel absorbed over a million Jewish refugees from both Europe and the Arab states. Israel would share hegemony with American Jewry and would begin to generate its own, unique Jewish customs and traditions, including reviving Hebrew as a primary spoken tongue – 2,000 years after it was previously used as the language of Jews during the biblical and Rabbinic periods.

Beliefs and practices

General

Judaism is a system of deed, not creed. Although Judaism does include a number of central tenets, its fundamental system is one of commanded actions, not commanded beliefs. Of the 613 commandments given in the Hebrew Bible, all are charges of behavior, not of faith or precept. Hence, Judaism is not a faith-system, as most Western religions are termed, but a system of commandments, or *mitzvot*. The *mitzvot* may be categorized as either ritual commandments or as ethical commandments. Examples of ritual commandments include observance of Shabbat (the Sabbath), animal sacrifice (in antiquity) for expiation of sins and guilt, dietary laws, and the obligation to circumcise eight-day-old boys. Examples of ethical commandments include honoring father and mother, leaving the corners of one's field for the hungry, not taking bribes, and respecting one's employees.

Despite this primary emphasis on behavior, beliefs are important. Judaism's fundamental belief is that God is one. Considered the central statement of Judaism, called the *Shema* (meaning: "Hear"), Deuteronomy 6:4 states, "Hear O Israel, Adonai is our God, Adonai is one." Judaism, therefore, is the first monotheistic religion and makes the singularity and uniqueness of God its chief theme. Rejection of any suggestion of multiple gods, or of the divisibility of God, is central to Judaism and distinguishes Judaism from other religions. The idea of the oneness of God was further developed by the twelfth-century Jewish philosopher and physician in Spain, Moses Maimonides, also known as the Rambam. Arguably, he was the greatest Jewish theologian and the most celebrated medieval medical practitioner. In his commentary on the Mishnah, Maimonides posited 13 principles of faith, asserting the existence, unity, incorporeality, and eternity of God – that God alone is to be worshipped and that God knows human behavior and metes reward and punishment, including the resurrection of the dead. Today, most Jews still adhere to the Rambam's initial principles, but far fewer accept the latter concepts.

A second essential precept of Judaism is the covenantal relationship (*brit*) between God and the people of Israel. God established the covenant with Abraham recorded in chapters 12 and 17 of Genesis, which declared that God would be God to the people of Israel, would bless them with plentiful progeny, and would give them the land of Canaan. For their part, the people would keep the commandments for every generation. The covenant would be renewed at Mount Sinai (Torah Exodus 19 and 20), and the symbol of the covenant would be the circumcision of the foreskin of all Jewish males.

Judaism professes values of the sanctity of life and respect for the body. Of all the commandments in the Torah, all except three of them (the prohibitions on murder, rape, and idolatry) may be violated for the sake of saving a life. This principle is called *piku'ah nefesh* (priority of saving a life). Existent life has priority over potential life. When necessary, a Jew may take risks for life, but is not required to risk his or her own life to save another. For instance, the Talmud discusses a situation when one may enter a burning building to save a life or the hypothetical case of travelers in the desert who must share a single flask of water. It teaches that one is not compelled to surrender oneself for the other. As well, because existent life has priority over potential life, when in conflict, the life of a pregnant mother takes precedence over that of the fetus. Judaism asserts the sanctity of the body, which is considered a sacred vessel of life and a gift from God. Thus, defacing the body, such as via tattoos or cutting, is prohibited as disrespect of God's gift. Likewise, Judaism also has disallowed autopsies or embalming, as each requires disfigurement of the body, and has formerly forbidden organ donation on the same grounds. Yet, after anti-rejection drugs, such as cyclosporine, have proven organ transplantation viable, rabbinic authorities have recanted their opposition on grounds of *piku'ah nefesh* – that for the sake of saving a life, the body of a deceased individual may be violated.

Judaism's festival sequence follows its particular, lunar calendar, with each day commencing and ending at sundown. Every seventh day at sunset, on Friday evening, commences *Shabbat* (the Sabbath), when Jews attend worship services at the synagogue and enjoy a festive *Shabbat* dinner. The Sabbath day, or Saturday, is a time of worship, study, rest, and family gathering. Key holy days include *Rosh Hashanah*, the Jewish New Year, and *Yom Kippur*, the Day of Atonement on which Jews fast to atone for misdeeds; these are the High Holy Days which occur in the early fall. The three biblical agricultural festivals of *Sukkot* (the fall harvest festival), Passover (*Pesach*, marking the exodus from Egypt), and *Shavuot* (commemorating the receipt of Torah at Sinai) are the major seasons of Jewish life and are treated as sacred days when the Jew abstains from work and worships in the synagogue. The eight-day winter celebration of Chanukah and the one-day spring festival of Purim mark Jewish victories over oppressors and include special foods. As well at Chanukah, Jews kindle an eight-branched candelabrum for eight nights. Besides *Yom Kippur*, there are other fast days in the Jewish calendar, most notably *Tisha B'Av*, which marks the destruction of the ancient temples. Out of mournfulness, Jews refrain from eating on such days. Also, Passover includes its own dietary restrictions, forbidding leavened foodstuffs and most grain products for the festival's eight days.

Kashrut (meaning "fit") is the name of the Jewish dietary system. Foodstuffs which are deemed proper for eating are called *kosher*, and those which are disallowed are termed *treif* (meaning "torn," i.e., the animal was killed by a predator and found in a field "torn"). Generally, animals whose meat is allowed are those mammals which chew their cud and have cloven, split hoofs. Hence, cattle and goats are allowed and are *kosher*, while pigs and dogs are disallowed. Permissible fish are those which have both fins and scales. Thus, catfish, which lack scales, and shellfish, which lack fins, are forbidden. Regarding fowl, the Torah lists those birds which are *kosher* and those which are *treif*, though basically predators and birds which eat carrion are *treif*. Also, in elucidating the Torah's laws of *kashrut*, the rabbis of the Talmud forbade mixing meat and milk in any individual meal. Thus, a cheeseburger or drinking milk with a chicken dish is *treif*. Some misinterpret the laws of *kashrut*, arguing that the rationale for these ancient precepts is concern for cleanliness and health. Although one may rightly argue that many of the forbidden animals may be unclean and may likely propagate disease, there is no evidence that such concerns prompted the Torah, or the Talmudic rabbis, to issue their restrictions. Rather, the laws of *kashrut* provide a discipline for Jewish living.

The Jewish life cycle consists of rituals which guide the Jew from the cradle to beyond the grave. Eight days after birth, a male Jewish child is entered into the covenant of Abraham through the procedure of circumcision (*brit milah*, "covenant of circumcision") at which the foreskin of the penis is surgically removed. Traditionally, a trained circumciser (*mohel*) would conduct the ritual in the home or in the synagogue, though today some parents opt to have the procedure performed in the hospital by a physician. At age 13, the ceremony of Bar or Bat Mitzvah ("son or daughter of the commandment") is conducted, at which the child leads the synagogue in worship and reads the Torah in Hebrew, demonstrating a competence in Jewish life. The final life cycle portal is death, on which more is addressed later in this chapter.

Lastly, there are two values which underlie and influence core Jewish practices: a commitment to cleanliness and a duty to modesty. By *halacha* (Jewish law), the Jew is required to wash one's hands at least seven times daily, including in the morning upon awakening, before eating, and upon touching any matter which is considered unclean. In the year 1348, for instance, when the Black Death pandemic devastated Europe with the bubonic plague, killing up to 50 percent of the general populace, the plague's incidence in Jewish communities was only a fraction of that elsewhere because Jews washed their hands regularly, thus defeating the spread of the disease. (Ironically, to explain how Jews were lesser affected by the plague, calumnious charges were propagated that Jews had caused the outbreak by poisoning the wells. Widespread oppression of Jews resulted.) Modesty (*tzniyut*) especially guides interaction between genders, principally in the Orthodox community. Among the Orthodox who are most observant of *halacha*, unmarried men and women do not touch, and a married man is not to touch or have any contact with women other than those of his immediate family. This limitation may cause Jewish women to seek female care providers when seeking medical treatment, though this would be suspended in life-threatening situations because of *piku'ah nefesh*. As well, among those who are observant of *halacha*, a woman will not have sexual relations with her husband while she is menstruating and is ritually unclean, and for one week thereafter.

Health and disease

Central to health beliefs within Judaism is that the body is a vessel which is a gift from God and is not to be violated. As such, the corollary also is true: that the physician has an obligation to heal and to return the condition of health to the ailing patient. Maimonides, the medieval Jewish physician and philosopher, taught in his code of Jewish law that the physician who withholds his services is considered as shedding blood (Maimonides *Yoreh De'ah* 336:1). This duty is derived from the biblical command, "You shall love your neighbor as yourself" (Torah Leviticus 19:18). Yet, there is a theological conflict in this charge to engage in the human art of healing. Namely, should one posit that all health and illnesses are ultimately derived from God, who is the source of life and of the natural order of the universe, the physician's intercession on behalf of healing represents a contravention and even an indictment of the divine system. By what right may the healthcare provider apply knowledge and skill and potentially breach the normal flow of health and illness? The Talmudic rabbis struggled with this concept yet argued that just as the soap-maker creates soap to facilitate cleaning and the farmer uses fertilizer to stimulate plant growth, so too a physician may employ the healing arts to engender healing. "Drugs and medicaments are the fertilizer and the physician is the tiller of the soil" (Eisenstein 1915: 581).

An early health belief which governed biblical practices was a profound regard for blood and bodily fluids. The Torah regarded blood as the life source and life force of both human and animal beings. Thus, among the laws of *kashrut* is the removal of blood from meat (see Torah Leviticus 17:10, 19:26). For human health, the ancient priest was to inspect bodily discharges and skin ailments for discoloration, and a person with such a discharge was rendered impure and sequestered until the person was deemed fit to be readmitted. Though greatly discussed in the Torah, these matters no longer govern modern Jewish life.

As described earlier, although circumcision, regard for cleanliness and modesty, and attention to *kashrut* are each general Judaic practices, each also may be construed as health practices. Circumcision certainly requires the trained hand of the circumciser, use of the proper implements, respect for cleanliness in healing, and the sensitive care of family to palliate the attendant suffering of the week-old infant. Although circumcision is a ritual practice, it surely is one of the earliest prescribed and regulated surgical procedures in human society, dating back to the patriarchal period (early to mid-second millennium BCE). Cleanliness, though initially charged as a social and ritual concern, may also be understood today as a matter of personal and social hygiene. Similarly, insofar as modesty unwittingly regulates human contact, it also may serve a social hygiene consideration by limiting the transfer of disease. These two concerns, cleanliness and limiting human contact, proved to be significant during the COVID-19 pandemic. Lastly, *kashrut* originally served to differentiate the Jewish community from others and to provide discipline to Jewish daily life. Later research clearly demonstrated that many proscribed animals carry disease, and that cleanliness adds a health element to the otherwise basic routines of life.

Among the principal commandments in Judaism is *bikur cholim* (visiting the sick). Although not expressly commanded in the Torah, the law is derived by the Talmudic rabbis from God visiting Abraham in the days following the patriarch's self-administered circumcision at the age of 99 (Torah Genesis 17:24, 18:1). The Talmud states, "As God clothes the naked, you clothe the naked. The Holy One visits the sick, as it is written, 'And God appeared to him (Abraham); so you visit the sick'" (BT *Sotah* 14a). Visiting the sick acts as a restorative deed, the rabbis taught. As God has implanted within every human being the image of God, which illness subverts, the visitor at the bedside reaffirms that divine value. Two thousand years ago, "Rabbi Acha bar Chanina taught, 'Whoever visits a sick person takes away one-sixtieth of his suffering'" (BT *Nedarim* 39b). Elsewhere in the Talmud, *bikur cholim* is considered one of the ten chief ethical commandments, the fulfillment of which is unlimited, and which yields fruit for all eternity (BT *Shabbat* 127a).

Lastly, within consideration of health practices it is worthy to note that Jewish teachings regarding sexual behavior and sexual mores affect both communal and individual health. In its table of prohibited relations, the Torah forbids marital and thus sexual unions between close members of the family (Torah Leviticus 18). Surely, the Torah was unaware of genetic science and the risk of an overly homogeneous genetic pool on the healthy diversity of the population. Proscribed unions likely were banned out of a sense of social morality and family probity. Yet, this also served to diversify the gene pool in an early stage of social development, thus promoting healthier progeny. Procreation clearly is the intent of sexual relations in the Torah, as evidenced in God's first communication to Adam, "Be fruitful and multiply" (Torah Genesis 1:28). Later, Maimonides would add the elements of pleasure and fulfillment as benefits of sexuality. Regulations, however, governed the sexual instinct. The woman was restricted from coitus while menstruating, and the Torah forbade the destruction of male seed – hence, male masturbation. Talmudic and later rabbinic commentators deliberated over permitted and prohibited means of contraception, though it is clear from the Talmud that contraception itself was allowed, and even required in certain circumstances. A nursing mother, for instance, must refrain from conceiving lest she wean her child prematurely, resulting in death (BT *Yebamot* 12b). Today, there are differences of opinion regarding the use of contraceptives within the Orthodox Jewish community, as precoital and postcoital devices may waste or destroy semen, thus conflicting with the prohibition. For all Jews, and especially more observant Jews, the use of oral contraceptives is less objectionable on *halachic* grounds and is even referenced in the Talmud when the wife of an early rabbi used a potion to render her sterile (BT *Yevamot* 65b). Currently, birth control procedures are commonplace in the Jewish community, except among the ultra-Orthodox.

There are a few diseases which, in the Jewish community, are commonly known as "Jewish genetic diseases," including Tay-Sachs disease, Gaucher disease type 1, Bloom's disease, familial dysautonomia, cystic fibrosis, and more recently breast and ovarian cancer. These illnesses appear in subsets of the Jewish community far more prevalently than in the general population and are recognized as genetic disorders occurring in Ashkenazic Jewish families from Eastern Europe. Due to social and religious conditions which prevailed for many centuries, the genetic mutations which resulted in these diseases became concentrated in this population, such that presently one in five Ashkenazic Jews may be a carrier of a gene for a threatening condition, according to the Jewish Genetic Disease Consortium. Today, many Jewish couples are encouraged to undergo genetic screening prior to marriage to determine if they are carriers of a mutation, and, if they are carriers, to consider amniocentesis and fetal monitoring during potential pregnancy.

Recent studies also have shown that the genetic mutations known as BRCA1 and BRCA2, which predispose one toward hereditary breast or ovarian cancer, occur inordinately in Ashkenazic Jewish women and men. For Jewish women who carry BRCA1, the mutation accounts for 16 percent of breast cancers and 39 percent of ovarian cancers, compared with 4 percent and 12 percent, respectively, in the general population. Moreover, in families with a history of breast or ovarian cancer, those in the Jewish community who carry the mutation have an 80–90 percent lifetime risk of breast cancer and a 40–50 percent lifetime risk of ovarian cancer. For Jewish men, carrying these mutations increases their risks for certain cancers, notably prostate cancer and male breast cancer. These data raise significant ethical and medical considerations, including concerns for prophylactic mastectomies, limited child-bearing windows, potential curative genetic engineering, insurability, and the welfare of one's children or grandchildren (Dorff 2003: 156; Rosner & Bleich 1987: 178; Bleich 1981: 103; Ford et al. 1994: 692–695; Struewing et al. 1995: 198–200; Kohn 2008: 14–21).

Turning to some prominent bioethical issues that impact all religions, Jewish tradition views life as beginning at birth – when the first breath of the newborn is inhaled. Life does not begin at conception. In fact, the Hebrew word for "soul" and for "breathing" are linked, *nefesh*, demonstrating that a soul is a breathing being. Thus, in the discussion regarding abortion, Judaism bears a distinct religious position. It asserts that since life commences with the newly born infant breathing independently of the mother, then abortion represents feticide – the destruction of a fetus – not infanticide, the killing of a human child's life. Yet, in the millennia of Jewish life, there have been varying opinions.

The Torah describes an incident in which a miscarriage occurs:

> When men fight, and one of them pushes a pregnant woman and a miscarriage results, but no other damage ensues, the one responsible shall be fined according as the woman's husband may exact from him, the payment to be based on reckoning.
>
> (Torah Exodus 21:22)

This verse demonstrates that the Torah considers the loss of a fetus not to be a capital offense. Potential life is not equivalent to an actual life. Rather, the fetus is considered as any other body part of the woman which may suffer injury in an accident, and for which pecuniary compensation for damages is determined by a judge. Later rabbinic interpretation in the Mishnah (Mishnah *Oholot* 7:6) affirmed that the life of the mother takes precedence over that of the fetus. This was further confirmed by Maimonides in his code of Jewish law (Maimonides *Hilchot Rotzeach* 1:9), though Maimonides added a caveat that the fetus may be destroyed because it is equivalent to an aggressor (*rodef*) which pursues and threatens the mother. Elsewhere, Jewish law details parameters of the *rodef*, delimiting the privileges of one who is threatened and respecting certain rights even of the aggressor. For instance, a homeowner at night may defend the family against an intruder and use deadly force assuming that the *rodef* is armed. However, during daylight the homeowner is not allowed to use such force unless the severity of the threat can be verified. Applying this line of Jewish legal reasoning, a pregnant woman may only abort the fetus when the pregnancy represents a significant danger to her life or well-being. Unresolved in Jewish thought are the limits to that threat: Is psychological or economic peril sufficient to justify abortion? Must there be a threat to life, or may it constitute a danger to the woman's well-being? These questions have not been decided definitively and are left to each individual's perspective on Judaism and ethics. There are those, especially in the Orthodox community, who argue that all forms of human life are sacred, including that in a test tube. Hence, they oppose all but necessary therapeutic abortions as infanticide. In the Progressive Jewish communities, the common interpretation is that the woman's rights take precedence over those of the potential life of the fetus and that abortion is a personal choice.

Regarding euthanasia and physician-assisted suicide, Judaism begins with the conviction, above all, that life is sacred. It is a gift from God and actually does not belong to human beings. Rather, humans are stewards of the life which is given. However, in the Mishnah, the rabbis taught, "Against your will you live, and against your will you die" (Mishnah *Pirkei Avot* 4:22). Yet, how much will is one free to exercise over the timeframes of one's life? When the conditions of life include exceptionally difficult suffering, may one choose to terminate life? Moreover, heeding the dictum of Ecclesiastes, which teaches that there is naturally, by divine design, "a time for being born and a time for dying" (Ketuvim Ecclesiastes 3:2), may one self-arrogate the decision as to when is the "time for dying"? Conversely, when it appears that the time for dying is nigh, may one hasten that time, or remove impediments which are sustaining life and thereby preventing the time for dying from asserting itself?

Judaism recognizes that there are two varieties of euthanasia, active and passive. Active euthanasia is an unjustified form of killing and is prohibited. Passive euthanasia, however, raises further questions. Modern medical technology can greatly prolong the life of a dying person and even sustain one who otherwise would have died. Is it permissible by Jewish teachings to disconnect that apparatus and to allow the person to expire naturally? Or is one duty-bound to undertake all measures, even extreme, to protect and prolong life?

The story of the death of an exalted sage of the Mishnah is illustrative. The sage, called "Rabbi" due to his lofty standing, was dying, and his disciples gathered around his bedside to pray that God would allow Rabbi further life. Seeing that her master was suffering and agitated by the prayers of his students, Rabbi's handmaid threw an earthen jug to the ground where it burst with a great noise. The disciples were startled and momentarily ceased their prayers. In that quiet instant, Rabbi's soul departed (BT *Ketubot* 104a). Interestingly, the Talmud does not censure the handmaid, but rather authorizes the episode.

This vignette offers an early example of passive euthanasia. Rabbi was dying, and the prayers of his students were comparable to life-support equipment in a modern hospital; they were an impediment to Rabbi's dying process. The maid opted to "unplug" the equipment and to allow Rabbi to die. The death of Rabbi, arguably the Mishnah's greatest figure, serves to validate passive euthanasia. Yet it also sets conditions for its permissibility. Judaism forbids any directly euthanizing action which prompts death, but for the *goses* (moribund patient) it sets no obligation to continue treatment or to prolong life. As such, removal of artificial nutrition or hydration is treated similarly, as it allows the course of death to continue. As well, quality of life is not the determining factor. The death of Rabbi occurred not to palliate a quality-of-life concern, but rather to remove an impediment to an imminent death.

The question of physician-assisted suicide follows similar reasoning. The physician is charged with prolonging life as well as with finding cures. Any action which actively hastens death is unjustifiable. Yet should death be looming, the physician is not obliged to extend life. However, what of the case of one who is suffering so mightily that he cries out, "Let me die"? May the physician heed his demands and assist him in ending his life? Jewish law also forbids suicide and treats it as unjustified killing (though to mitigate the anguish on mourners, the rabbis determined to treat suicide as an accident). Assisting one to commit suicide, therefore, is the same as abetting a murder and is not allowed. Clearly, however, physicians are stirred by the compelling moral desire to mollify pain and bring comfort to suffering patients. Jewish law does not prohibit a physician from prescribing strong analgesic medications such as morphine to control pain, though it may concurrently suppress respiratory function and allow the process of dying to proceed. Palliative care is understood in Judaism as proper and necessary, yet it must be managed carefully when death is near. In 1997, the Conservative Movement's Committee on Jewish Law and Standards issued a ruling which stated, "Patients and their caregivers ... have the tradition's permission to withhold or withdraw impediments to the natural process of dying ..." (Dorff 2003: 376).

Regarding gender, Judaism makes no distinction either in the value of life or in treatment based on the gender of the patient. All life is of equal value. Similarly, there is no gender limitation as to who may work in healthcare fields. Of concern, as discussed earlier, is regard for *tzniyut* (modesty). Primarily in the Orthodox community, women must have the option to see female healthcare providers so as not to risk violating this precept.

There is much current discussion regarding gender identity, with consideration for those who identify in other than the traditional binary male or female categories. Two thousand years ago, the Talmud (Mishnah, *Bikkurim 4:1*) recognized six different gender definitions, including male and female, the *androgynos*, or hermaphrodite; the *tumtum*, the one with underdeveloped genitalia; the *eylonit* (the feminine man); and the *saris* (the masculine woman). Today, these categories and others require the religious and medical communities to continue to stretch their respective boundaries to protect the mental, physical, and spiritual well-being of those who seek care in their gender identities and mental health.

The COVID-19 pandemic has raised consideration of both vaccination and public health policy. Orthodox Jewish tradition and rabbinic scholars, since the advent of vaccinations in the eighteenth century, have advocated vaccination. Their vital reasoning stems from the concern that physicians have a charge to heal the sick, but may they do so by sickening the healthy? Supporting vaccination, they subscribed to tenets of Jewish law which assert that it is reasonable to put oneself in a modest risk (potentially making the healthy person ill) for the sake of securing the well-being of the greater whole. Moreover, the Talmud (BT *Shabbat* 129a) teaches that for one who is ill, but not in life-threatening danger, the benefit of taking action outweighs the risks. Modern teachers (Bleich) argue that to be unvaccinated was religiously irresponsible. Similarly, those of progressive streams of Jewish life have followed the Talmudic dictum of *dina d'malchuta dina* (BT *Baba Batra* 54b), the law of the land is the law of the land; all citizens have an obligation to follow secular governmental laws where they apply, including in public health concerns (Muravsky et al. 2021).

Death and dying

In the Book of Ecclesiastes, one reads the famous poem, "A season is set for everything, a time for every experience under heaven: A time for being born and a time for dying" (Ketuvim Ecclesiastes 3:1–2). Death, therefore, is considered a natural part of the flow of life, and certainly in earlier days it was a regular experience of adults and children alike. The Torah records that, upon death, each of the patriarchs "was gathered to his kin" (Torah Genesis 25:17, 35:29, 49:33). Natural death occurred in the family chambers, not in hospitals or nursing facilities where today death is moderated, mitigated, and euphemized. Thus, in understanding and respecting death and treating it as the portal to the great mystery of beyond, Judaism also imbued death and dying with very practical, intimate, and earthly boundaries and protocols.

A person, near death, is called a *goses* (moribund). This is not a medically technical definition, but rather defines the patient who is in a persistent and deteriorating non-responsive condition. This description heralds the expected close of life. In Jewish tradition, life begins at the first breath in accordance with the second creation story in Genesis. Describing the creation of man in the Garden of Eden, Torah recounts, "He (God) blew into his nostrils the breath of life, and man became a living being" (Torah Genesis 2:7). As such, classical Jewish thinking held that life's parameters begin and end with breathing – when the soul enters and departs from the body. Thus, death occurs with the cessation of breathing. The rabbis prescribe taking much care to be certain that breathing has ceased, and that death has occurred, even waiting half an hour before removing the body from the deathbed. Liturgically, it is a custom that the dying person, or a surrogate if not capable, recites a final prayer of forgiveness as death approaches.

Because Jewish funeral procedures were designed in the ancient Near East in days before refrigeration and because Jewish law prohibits defacing the body (hence, disallowing embalming), burial was to occur expeditiously once death is confirmed – that is, within 24 hours, if possible. Thus, today there may be pressure on the physician to swiftly complete the necessary certification to allow the family and the funeral professionals to arrange for a timely burial. Respecting Jewish law, which dictates that the body is a sacred vessel of life, the body is not to be left alone. Observant Jews will arrange for a *shomeir* (a watchman) to sit with the body in the funeral establishment until it is prepared for burial and to recite words of the Psalms. As well, in keeping with tradition of not disfiguring the body, cremation was disallowed, although today some will opt for cremation. Historically, for the same reasons, autopsies were prohibited, except where municipal statutes require them.

Similarly, organ transplantation presented significant difficulties. *Piku'ah nefesh*, the primacy of saving a life, allows one to suspend or violate most Jewish laws in order to save a life. Yet, in the early days of organ transplantation, the procedure often resulted in both the death of the donor and of the recipient and defacing the donor's body. Thus, in the 1960s, rabbinic authorities deemed that transplantation risked greater hazards than were allowed and concluded that organ transplantation was tantamount to murder, thus was impermissible. Only with new drugs which suppressed the immune system, granting the recipient a realistic chance at survival, did the leading Orthodox medical ethicists consent to organ transplantation. As well, with the publication of the Ad Hoc Committee of Harvard Medical School to Examine the Definition of Death in 1968, offering an understanding of death not only as the loss of cardiorespiratory function, but also neurological death upon a flat electroencephalogram, did the Orthodox join the Progressive Jewish communities in accepting the permissibility of organ transplantation (Dorff 2003: 229–232). Presently, motivated by the Jewish ethics of fixing the world and saving lives, many synagogues conduct donor promotions, encouraging congregants to register as potential donors.

The Jewish funeral is not theological. Its primary purpose is to guide and support the mourners to manage their difficult process of grieving and balancing their lives anew, rather than to usher the soul of the deceased into eternity. Admittedly, the mystery of what is beyond death compels the Jew and the non-Jew alike, yet Judaism is steeped in commandments which guide the Jew to live in the present world. Thus, the Jewish funeral is often brief and relatively lacking in pageantry. Sharing memories and expressing care for the bereaved are the central components of the funeral.

Conclusion

Judaism, and Jews, have a long history and regard for health and healing. Similarly, Jewish sacred texts and *halacha*, Jewish law, include much instruction addressing practice and values which govern medical behavior and ethics. Originating in the Hebrew Bible and continuing through each successive stratum of Jewish legal literature, including the Mishnah, Talmud, and codes of the great philosophers and codifiers such as Moses Maimonides, central precepts such as the sanctity of life and respect for the body have always informed Jewish life and stimulated great attention to the healing arts. Thus, healthcare considerations are not secondary or tertiary within the Jewish religious

Table 11.1 Dos and don'ts

Dos	Don'ts
1. Be sensitive to the Jewish festival calendar and holy days which have specific expectations or limitations.	1. One should kindly refrain from offering "theological explanations" of death to a bereaved Jewish family member.
2. Be respectful of the dietary concerns of kashrut. Besides making available *kosher* foods for the hospitalized Jewish patient, awareness of particular dietary considerations due to festival customs also would be advised.	2. One ought to be careful in touching – even offering a courtesy handshake – to an Orthodox Jew of the opposite gender. Thus, medically unnecessary contact ought to be resisted, and one should not be insulted if, when offering a handshake as an introduction in a hospital room, it is not accepted, or is rebuffed.
3. It is always encouraged that a rabbi or Jewish chaplain, where available, be informed when a Jewish patient is in the hospital.	3. Be careful not to assume that a Jewish patient is either Orthodox or not Orthodox merely by his or her appearance. It may be wise to inquire if there are any religious considerations to be respected.
4. When possible, endeavor to be expeditious when managing certification of death of a Jewish person, to allow for a timely funeral.	

system; rather they bear a central position in Judaism and compel basic ethics. Witness the inordinate number of Jews in the healing professions, which has been evident in every generation and in every region wherever Jews have resided. And, despite vast diversity in religious beliefs among adherents of different streams of Judaism, the Jewish world has built largely progressive positions on controversial ethical matters such as abortion, euthanasia, and organ transplantation. These positions are based on consideration for existent life over potential life, concern for the dignity of the patient, and most importantly, the primary ethos of saving life at all costs. Furthermore, in raising behaviors such as diet, cleanliness, and modesty to religious precepts, Judaism also instituted social hygiene as a sacred principle. In all, healthcare considerations are basic and fundamental to Judaism and to the Jewish people.

Case study #1

The use of arts and crafts in the profession of occupational therapy grew out of the arts and crafts movement at the end of the nineteenth century. Occupational therapists use a variety of media, games, arts, and crafts to rehabilitate patients. This is no different for the pediatric population, as the primary occupation of children is to play and engage in crafts.

Mignon, a 7-year-old girl, had hypotonia and frequent elbow dislocations due to ligament laxity. She presented with overall low tone in her trunk/core and upper extremities. Mignon and one of her parents attended therapy sessions weekly. She worked on increasing upper extremity strength as well as weight bearing tasks, designed to increase upper body and arm strength.

At the initial evaluation, I learned that I was working with a family who identified with the Jewish tradition and the child attended a local private Jewish school. I grew up in Florida with Jewish neighbors, so I was somewhat familiar with Jewish holiday customs. During the holidays, I like to have seasonally appropriate crafts and themed activities. I had gathered materials for constructing paper Christmas trees and other Christmas coloring sheets, but I didn't want to offer those to this child, so I looked up Hanukkah crafts and had alternate options for this child throughout the season. One craft was making a Chanukah Menorah (candelabrum) from popsicle sticks. The child and her mother were really surprised and appreciated that I had selected options just for her.

Questions for reflection

1. Sensing the dissonance of Christmas holiday toys for a Jewish family requires a knowledge of Jewish beliefs and holidays. Where does the average American pick up this information, if at all?
2. Traditionally, Hanukkah was considered a minor Jewish holiday, but it has recently grown in importance among American Jews, including the sharing of presents with children. What factors might have contributed to this growing importance even among secular Jews?
3. In your chosen profession what are the possible small tokens or gestures toward patients and their families rendered in response to their religious sensibilities outside the norm?

Submitted by Angela Sampson

Case study #2

A 70-year-old Orthodox Jewish female presented to a hospital ED during the afternoon of *Kol Nidre*, preceding the day of Yom Kippur. The patient was very distressed by potentially being hospitalized and requested to be seen as soon as possible with the hope that she would be discharged sufficiently before sunset, early enough to participate in *Kol Nidre* services. The patient's nurse was moved by this patient's commitment and felt concerned that the patient was not home with her family preparing for Yom Kippur.

The nurse advocated for the team to see her as quickly as possible. After two hours, the nurse approached the attending physician again and reiterated that this patient needed to be seen quickly. The doctor became upset and said that other patients had waited longer and that she had more critical patients that she needed to prioritize, and that this patient's condition was not life-threatening.

Questions for reflection

1. Why is Yom Kippur so important among Jewish holidays? Why was the approaching sunset an issue?
2. Should the team prioritize treating this patient in anticipation of the Holy Day? Why or why not?
3. If the Jewish patient was treated ahead of patients who had been waiting even longer, how might the nurse address their complaints?
4. How could the nurse further support this patient in her religious observance if the patient was unable to leave the hospital? What other members of the interdisciplinary team could she involve?

*Submitted by Joset Brown

Glossary

Cantor or Hazzan The Cantor is the officiant who sings the Jewish liturgy during worship (male or female).
Erev Shabbat This term refers to the time on Friday evening just prior to sunset when the Sabbath is about to begin.
Fleischig The Yiddish term used to describe a meat-based meal.
Milchig The Yiddish term used to describe a dairy-based meal.
Parve The Yiddish term used to describe a meal which is neutral, neither dairy nor meat.
Rabbi or Rav The terms used to refer to the religious leader of Jews (male or female).
Shabbat or Shabbes The Sabbath Day, Friday evening to Saturday evening.
Siddur The Jewish prayer book.
Synagogue, Temple, or Shul The facility or building of Jewish worship and study.
Torah The scroll of the Five Books of Moses.

Note

1 All quotations from the Hebrew scriptures, Torah and Ketuvim, are translations of the author.

Bibliography

Babylonian Talmud (n. d.), www.sefaria.org/texts/Talmud

Bleich, JD. (1981) *Judaism and Healing: Halachic Perspectives*. New York: Ktav Publishing House.

DellaPergola, S. (2021) *American Jewish Yearbook, 2022*. Springer Nature. https://link.springer.com/chapter/10.1007/978-3-030-99750-2_8

Dorff, EN. (2003) *Matters of Life and Death: A Jewish Approach to Modern Medical Ethics*. Philadelphia: The Jewish Publication Society.

Eisenstein, JD. (ed.) (1915) *Otzar Midrashim*, vol. 2. New York: Mishor.

Ford, D., Easton, DF., Bishop, DT., Narod, SA., and Goldgar, DE. (1994) "Risks of Cancer in BRCA1-Mutation Carriers," *Lancet, 343*: 692–695.

Greenberg, S., and Levine, JD. (eds) (1978) *Mahzor Chadash: The New Mahzor*. Bridgeport, CT: Media Judaica.

Jewish Agency for Israel (2022) "Jewish Population Rises to 15.3 Million Worldwide, with Over 7 Million Residing in Israel." www.jewishagency.org/jewish-population-rises-to-15-3-million-worldwide-with-over-7-million-residing-in-israel/

Jewish Virtual Library, AICE (2022) "Total Jewish Population in the United States." www.jewishvirtuallibrary.org/jewish-population-in-the-united-states-nationally

Kohn, DJ. (ed.) (2008) *Life, Faith, and Cancer: Jewish Journeys Through Diagnosis, Treatment, and Recovery*. New York: URJ Press.

Maimonides (n. d.), a. Hilchot Rotzeach. Eliyahu Touger, translator. https://www.sefaria.org/Mishneh_Torah%2C_Murderer_and_the_Preservation_of_Life.1.9?lang=bi&with=all&lang2=enb. Yoreh De'ah, in Shulchan Arukh. Joseph Karo. https://www.sefaria.org/Shulchan_Arukh%2C_Yoreh_De'ah.336?lang=bi

Mishnah (n. d.), www.sefaria.org/texts/Mishnah

Muravsky, NL., Betesh, GM., and McCoy, RG. (2021) "Religious Doctrine and Attitudes Toward Vaccination in Jewish Law," *Journal of Religion and Health*, October 27, 2021: 1–16.

Pew Research Center (2020) "Jewish Americans in 2020." www.pewforum.org/2021/05/11/jewish-americans-in-2020/

Rosner, F., and Bleich, JD. (eds) (1987) *Jewish Bioethics*. New York: Hebrew Publishing.

Struewing, JP., Abeliovich, D., Perez, T., Avishai, N., Kaback, MM., Collins, FS., and Brody, LC. (1995) "The Carrier Frequency of the BRCA1 185delAG Mutation is Approximately 1 Percent in Ashkenazi Jewish Individuals," *Nature Genetics, 11*: 198–200.

12 Christianity

David R. Larson

For God so loved the world that he gave his only son, so that everyone who believes in him may not perish but have eternal life.

(John 3:16)[1]

He said to him, "you shall love the Lord your God with all your heart, and with all your soul, and with all your mind." This is the greatest and first commandment. And a second is like it: "You shall love your neighbor as yourself." On these two commandments hang all the law and the prophets.

(Matthew 22:37–40)

Introduction

Christianity is the largest and most widely dispersed religion in the world today. It is also the most diverse, especially when it comes to health and healing. On the one hand, its healing methods can be simple, unsophisticated, and some say superstitious. On the other hand, everywhere Christians have gone they have established excellent medical institutions to help humankind deal with illness and disease.

Some may find it difficult to see much similarity between "faith healing" meetings before hundreds and sometimes thousands of awe-struck people gathered in public places like gymnasiums, stadiums, and tents, on the one hand, and the quiet scientific activity of Christian institutions that treat sick people with resources such as chemotherapy, organ transplantation, and proton beam accelerators. These differences are real and significant. But they are all part of the Christian story.

Demographics

About one third (31%) of all the people in the world are Christians. Virtually all Christians belong to one of its three main branches: Roman Catholicism, Orthodoxy, Protestantism (Pew Research Center 2012; Pew Research Center 2017). Roman Catholics are the most numerous, at approximately 50%, and Protestants are the second largest at 37%. Both Roman Catholicism and Protestantism have cultural roots in the Latin west. Roman Catholicism is global, tightly organized, and led by the Pope from the Vatican, their historical center in Rome, Italy. There are thousands of Protestant denominations and an uncountable number of independent congregations and smaller groups. Orthodox

DOI: 10.4324/9781003288862-12

Christian groups (Eastern or Russian for instance) are third in number at 12%. Their cultural roots tie them more closely to Greece and Eastern influences. Orthodox Christians are organized in regional, self-governing churches.

In the United States, down sharply over the past several decades, roughly 63% report being Christian. Almost 30% now report they are unaffiliated with any particular religion (Pew Research Center 2022; Public Religion Research Institute 2021). Adherents to non-Christian religions such as Judaism, Hinduism, Buddhism, and Islam make up the rest at roughly 7% (American Demografia 2022; Statista 2021).

About one fifth (20%) of the Christians who live in the United States today are Roman Catholics. There are three groups of Protestants in the United States. The Mainline Protestants amount to about one seventh of the population (15%) (American Demografia 2022). Their largest denominations are the: United Methodist Church, Evangelical Lutheran Church in America, Episcopal Church, Presbyterian Church (USA), American Baptist Churches, United Church of Christ, and Disciples of Christ.

About one fourth (25%) of the Protestant Christians living in the US are Evangelical. Their largest denominations are the: Southern Baptist Convention, Churches of God in Christ, Assemblies of God, and Lutheran Church-Missouri Synod. Most Evangelical Protestants emerged from the revolt of the Fundamentalists in the early years of the twentieth century against the tendencies toward "modernism" in what are now the Mainline denominations.

The Historically Black Protestant Christians in the US are the smallest in number (6%) (American Demografia 2022). Their largest denominations are the: African Methodist Episcopal Church, African Methodist Episcopal Zion Church, Christian Methodist Episcopal Church, Church of God in Christ, National Baptist Convention of America, National Baptist Convention, USA, and the Progressive National Baptist Convention. These denominations comprise a somewhat different stream of Protestantism in the US which has its own subtly distinctive beliefs, practices, and ways of worshipping.

History

Born in Bethlehem and reared in Nazareth, as Christians remember it, Jesus left his carpenter shop as a young man and became a traveling preacher, teacher, and healer. His message was that the Kingdom or Reign of God was at hand and that in some ways it was already present. Like the Hebrew scriptures he had studied, he taught that true morality can be summarized in love for God and neighbor. Yet he emphasized the need for a way of life that was more inward, thoroughgoing, and inclusive.

Some political and religious leaders of the time took offense at Jesus' words and deeds, interpreting his emphasis upon God's Kingdom or Reign as a threat to their own. This is why Pontius Pilate, the primary representative of the Roman Empire which was occupying the land, had him tortured and then killed by crucifixion. Most Christians believe that on the third day after his death he was resurrected. After a brief time, he ascended to heaven with a promise someday soon to return in power and glory.

The first 500 years of Christian history were marked by rapid growth and increasing cultural influence. Emperor Constantine made Christianity the official religion of the Roman Empire in 323 CE. The first eight Ecumenical Councils convened between the fourth and ninth centuries. These were large and sometimes lengthy meetings of Christian leaders which clarified and made more widely spread basic Christian beliefs. Christians to this day frequently recite the "Creed," or summary of beliefs, which the Council of Nicaea made official in the fourth century (325 CE).

> I believe in one God, the Father Almighty, Maker of heaven and earth, and of all things visible and invisible. And in one Lord Jesus Christ, the only-begotten Son of God, begotten of the Father before all worlds; God of God, Light of Light, very God of very God; begotten, not made, being of one substance with the Father, by whom all things were made. Who, for us men and for our salvation, came down from heaven, and was incarnate by the Holy Spirit of the virgin Mary, and was made man; and was crucified also for us under Pontius Pilate; He suffered and was buried; and the third day He rose again, according to the Scriptures; and ascended into heaven, and sits on the right hand of the Father; and He shall come again, with glory, to judge the quick and the dead; whose kingdom shall have no end. And I believe in the Holy Ghost, the Lord and Giver of Life; who proceeds from the Father and the Son; who with the Father and the Son together is worshipped and glorified; who spoke by the prophets. And I believe one holy catholic and apostolic Church. I acknowledge one baptism for the remission of sins; and I look for the resurrection of the dead, and the life of the world to come. Amen.
>
> (*Nicene Creed*)

Roman Catholicism dominated in Western Europe for centuries, with the theologians Augustine of North Africa in the fifth century and Thomas Aquinas in Italy and France in the thirteenth century as the era's intellectual giants. Eastern Orthodoxy was far more influential in the Eastern part of the former Roman Empire. These two branches of Christianity officially split in 1055 CE and they are still divided.

History began to move away from Rome beginning with the Renaissance in fourteenth-century Italy. Tensions boiled over with the Protestant Reformation in the sixteenth century, pre-eminently with Martin Luther in Germany and John Calvin in Switzerland. Against what they perceived to be spiritual and administrative abuses of the Roman Catholic church, the reformers emphasized the authority of Scripture – as interpreted by individual Christians – against that of the church hierarchy, the centrality of salvation by God's grace (without any human participation), and the "priesthood" of all believers – that every Christian has received a calling from God for ministry and each calling is equally sacred.

The seventeenth century in Western Europe was beset by religious warfare. This contributed to the flowering of the European Enlightenment, which triggered the switch from pre-modern to modern ways of thinking and acting. Deism was one widespread response. Its naturalistic view of God and the universe eliminated much of Christianity in the name of human reason. This was the religion of Thomas Jefferson, Benjamin Franklin, and other American leaders. The Evangelical Revival in England and North America was a different response. Its leaders – principally John and Charles Wesley and George Whitefield from England and Jonathan Edwards in America – put more emphasis upon emotion, what Edwards called "the religious affections" (Edwards 1959).

The nineteenth century was as decisive for Christianity as the sixteenth and fourth had been. On the one hand, more skeptical ways of studying the Bible, the writings of Charles Darwin, Karl Marx and, later, Sigmund Freud and the arrival of many Roman Catholic immigrants challenged the basically Protestant nation as never before. In addition to all of its other devastating consequences, the American Civil War divided Christian denominations into "southern" and "northern" denominations that have long persisted. Well into the twenty-first century, for instance, there is still both the American (Northern) Baptists and the Southern Baptist Convention denominations.

On the other hand, the nineteenth century set forth the largest missionary endeavors in Christian history. The battle against slavery which Christians and others fought was a success. So were many reform movements which addressed the social evils of the time. The idea that they were leading a gradual development into what sounded like "heaven on earth" permeated many Christian circles. This was partly because those who had believed that the Second Coming of Jesus would occur on a certain date, and that they knew that date but were wrong, subsequently experienced a Great Disappointment ("Great Disappointment," 2023).

Many had accepted the views of William Miller who eventually settled on the date for the Second Coming of Jesus as October 22, 1844. When it did not occur, a few of them continued to meet and eventually they formed the Seventh-day Adventist denomination in which the writings of Ellen G. White continue to have much influence and authority. Joseph Smith founded the Church of Jesus Christ of Latter-Day Saints, or more simply, Latter Day Saints or even Mormons, in the nineteenth century. Charles Taze Russell founded the Jehovah's Witnesses and Mary Baker Eddy founded the Christian Scientists then as well. The next chapter of this book discusses all four of these in detail because each of them has beliefs which sometimes complicate the efforts of health care professionals to serve them.

In 1900 some Christian leaders took over a struggling journal and renamed it *Christian Century* because they believed that this was what the twentieth century would be. It became the leading journal for Mainline Protestants. Jesuits founded *America Magazine* in 1909 and it became the most widely read journal among Roman Catholics. Evangelist Billy Graham, in 1956, founded the journal *Christianity Today* as a conservative Protestant option. It became the most influential Evangelical journal.

In the first years of the twentieth century, the circulation of *Christian Century* was 36,000, *America Magazine* was 49,000, and *Christianity Today* was 136,000. This sums up as well as anything else what happened to Mainline Protestants in the twentieth century. They experienced a Great Disappointment of their own.

It is not difficult to see why. World War I, World War II, the Korean War, and the Viet Nam war chastened Christian optimism. So did the Spanish Flu, the Great Depression, and the Cold War. Many objected to the support Mainline Protestants gave to the Civil Rights movement and the liberation endeavors for persons of color, women, homosexuals, the handicapped, and the environment. Many thought that Mainline Protestants were too supportive of revolutionary movements abroad, especially those who were making use of some of Karl Marx's ideas. In the battle over abortion in the American Culture Wars they tended to be "pro-choice" when many thought they should be "pro-life." Many had the impression that Mainline Protestants had rejected many of Christianity's basic beliefs without replacing them with something better. Many Mainline Protestants today regret no longer being at the nation's cultural center. Many others are relieved to be pushed closer to its edges from which it can more successfully confront the social evils of our time.

A shift in priorities occurred in Mainline Protestants, Evangelicals, and Roman Catholic Christians the in the twentieth century. For its first 60 or so years, they were primarily concerned with their own inner lives. How to deal with anxiety, guilt, mean-inglessness, and the fear of death and similar things in order to have peace of mind was a primary concern. Although they were expressed in denominationally different ways, the answers Christian leaders gave were similar across all of them.

How to relate to society at large in a time of rapid change was the primary concern over the last 40 years. The earlier consensus on psychological issues crumbled before the political and economic issues they now faced. This opened up divisions between the Protestant denominations and within them. Roman Catholics managed these challenges somewhat more successfully; however, it also experienced internal tensions.

Although Roman Catholics had studied bioethical issues for centuries, this is when it became a professional "field" of its own with the typical conferences, publications, and institutes. The secular Hastings Center in New York and the Kennedy Institute of Bioethics at Roman Catholic Georgetown University in Washington, D.C. led the way in creating "think tanks," but others established similar organizations throughout the nation. Specialists called it a "field" rather than a "discipline" or "specialty" because it involved philosophers, theologians, lawyers, empirical and social scientists, humanities professors, as well as doctors, nurses, and other health care professionals. Eventually, though, "clinical ethics" did become a specialty on its own.

Throughout its long history, Christianity has made many contributions to theoretical and practical medicine. Yet it is impossible to distinguish the history of Western medicine from the history of Western Judaism, Christianity, and Islam. Although these are somewhat different streams, their waters intermingle so often and so deeply that no one can know where one begins and the other ends. What is more, the contributions of these religions to health and healing may reside more in what they believed than in what they did.

Beliefs and practices

Christian beliefs differ greatly in their details; however, if one stands back and considers them from a distance, they appear remarkably similar in their main outlines. Also, Christians share many convictions with Jews and Muslims. All three are *"Abrahamic"* religions because they each recount their formative narrative to the person and faith of the biblical personage, Abraham.

Like Jews and Muslims, Christians center their lives on the *one true God* who brought the universe into being and continues to sustain it. God is both immanent, within the universe, and transcendent, beyond and greater than it. There is no place where God is absent, nothing that can be known that God does not know, and nothing that can be done that God cannot do. Everything about God is worthy of admiration and acclaim. This is especially so of God's steadfast love that endures forever.

Most Christians believe that the one genuine *God is "Triune,"* though they do not believe in three Gods. Harkening back to the days when the same one actor *personified* different people by changing masks, they believe that the one God is at least for us three *persons*: Father, Son, and Holy Spirit. Some emphasize how similar these are and some, how different. Yet no true Christian is a tritheist. They are all triune monotheists. The word "substance" means "essence." The word "person" comes from the different masks or roles of actors in theatrical performances. "Perichoresis," or "dancing in a circle," instead of vertically or horizontally, is one metaphor Christians have used when thinking about the three members of the Trinity (the shorthand term for referring to the Triune God). One implication of this doctrine is that relationships characterize everything, from God to subatomic particles and smaller.

Although they vary in their emphasis, Christians believe that *God is revealed* in nature, history, experience, reason, scripture, and, most decisively, in Jesus Christ. Like Jews and Muslims, Christians are "people of the book." This book, the "Bible," is actually a "library" with material from many different times and places. Taken together, these documents from long ago tell a story. It is a story about God's interaction with people and other things. Christians believe that this story points to the direction in which our lives should move today.

The biblical idea of *creation* distinguishes Christian belief from at least two other alternatives. One of them is the kind of dualism that posits a deep, wide, and unbridgeable divide between the spiritual and physical realms of human life; the second is the kind of monism or pantheism that pictures the universe as a single whole, with all particular things and people as its partial expressions. Christians believe that dualism is too negative about the physical features of life and that monism or pantheism undervalues the relative individuality of each thing.

Christians believe that all human beings are created in the *"image of God,"* the expression coming from the biblical account of the creation of humankind. This does not mean that they look like God. It means that they share in a limited and imperfect way some of God's most important characteristics: reason, freedom, memory, anticipation, purposefulness, intimacy, and perhaps even laughter. Although other animals possess these characteristics in lesser or greater degrees, they characterize human life in a qualitatively superior way.

The basic idea of the Christian concept of *sin* is that pain, suffering, and evil are not essential elements of existence. "Intruders" and "violators," they are the global consequences of misusing the freedom God has given humankind. "Original sin" refers to the difficulties and inabilities all people inherit. "Actual sins" are the thoughts, words, and deeds in which they freely indulge even when they know they should not. Christians believe that everyone except Jesus Christ is a sinner.

They believe that human beings cannot extricate themselves from sin and its consequences: discord, guilt, meaninglessness, and death. This is something only God can do. The entire Bible is a story of how God has repeatedly done this for others and the assurance that God can do the same for people today. All religions have a story. For many of them, it is explanatory; for Christians it is essential. They believe that the story of *salvation* is the best of all narratives because it proclaims the good news that God loves unconditionally.

The word "Jesus" is a name, the word "*Christ*" a title. It conveys the meaning of the prior Hebrew words: "Messiah" or "Anointed." For Christians, Jesus Christ is the long-awaited Jewish "Messiah." He is "Immanuel," which is to say, "God with Us," when the word "Us" refers to everybody; all of humankind.

Christians believe that Jesus Christ was the incarnation of God, the embodiment of God in human life. In this sense, Jesus was truly human and truly God. When Christians talk of Jesus as the *"Son of God"* they do not mean that their relationship was like the biological one between human fathers and sons. They are speaking as the ancients did when describing God's reaction to the coronation of a new King. "This is my beloved son," or "This is my only begotten son," God said in praise of the new monarch. According to the biblical story, this is what God said of Jesus. Thus, "Son of God" is a relational term not a biological one.

From the very start it has been difficult for Christians to avoid confusion in their two-fold conviction that Jesus was *truly God and truly human*. One of the earliest problems was called "Docetism." It denied the true humanity of Jesus, holding that he only appeared to be human. "Arianism" eventually became a problem as well. It denied the true divinity of Jesus, picturing him as divine but not equal with God. There were many other similar challenges. In 451 CE, the Council of Chalcedon declared the following which has become known as he Chalcedon Creed:

> We confess that one and the same Christ, Lord, and only-begotten Son, is to be acknowledged in two natures without confusion, change, division, or separation. The distinction between natures was never abolished by their union, but rather the character proper to each of the two natures was preserved as they came together in one person and one hypostasis.
>
> (Chalcedon Creed 451 CE)

This settled the issue for most Christians, even if some have continued debating it ever since. In addition to Jesus' preaching, teaching, and healing, most Christians emphasize his *death and resurrection* and their special importance in freeing humans from sin and its negative consequences: discord, guilt, meaninglessness, and death. In trying to explain how this happens they have used various analogies, as the Bible itself does, and each reflects the social settings from which it emerges.

Maybe the process of *atonement* is like being found guilty in a court of law and having someone else pay the penalty or take the punishment. Or perhaps it is like being kidnapped and then being set free because someone else paid the ransom. Or could it be that the process is more like a school in which we learn about God's love when we concentrate on the final hours of Jesus' life, seeing how he chose to accept suffering than to inflict it upon others? Christians have used all these metaphors, and many others, claiming all along that the full process of atonement is beyond the capacity of mere words to describe.

Christians believe that the church is the "*body of Christ*," meaning that today it continues the preaching, teaching, and healing ministry of Jesus. Many apply it to Christians in all denominations; however, others restrict its usage to those they take to be genuine.

Christians differ in how they view the billions of people around the world who are *non-Christians*. Many hold that these persons cannot experience salvation because they have not decided to become followers of Jesus, and this is so even if they have never heard of him. Many others hold that God is equally at work in all the religions of the world and that their genuine adherents are all equally saved. Most Christians take one of many alternatives between these extremes. One of these "middle" alternatives holds that, even though God is at work in all religions, people who are active in ones other than Christianity can still benefit from hearing its "good news," and that Christians can benefit from hearing theirs.

Christian *worship and life* center upon rituals or practices signifying the presence of God in ordinary life called "sacraments." Roman Catholic and Eastern Orthodox Christians hold that there are seven: (1) *baptism*, the use of water to celebrate the beginning of a new Christian life, (2) *confirmation*, determining on the basis of further consideration to live as a Christian, (3) *matrimony*, the lifelong, loving, and sexually exclusive union of a man and woman who establish a Christian home, (4) *penance*, doing sometimes difficult things that provide discipline when it is needed, (5) *prayer for the sick*, asking God for strength and wisdom in the face of illness and death, (6) *holy orders*, the decision by some to live their entire lives in service to the church as priests, and (7) *communion* or the Eucharist, a celebration with bread and wine as emblems of the sacrificial body and blood of Jesus Christ, though some assert the bread and wine become his literal body and blood when offered as a sacrament. Most Protestant Christians practice only two of the seven sacraments: baptism and communion.

Just as they believe that Jesus Christ was resurrected from the grave, the majority of Christians hold that they will experience *life in the hereafter*. But again, they differ on the details. Most hold that the body and soul are so different that the soul does not die when the body does, and that instead the soul goes either to heaven, paradise, or to hell, punishment. Some contend that body and soul are inseparable, and that death includes the entire person, body, and soul alike. They do not even like to talk about "body *and* soul," as though they are basically different. They much prefer "embodied soul" or "in-souled body," or just plain "person." Both groups look forward to the resurrection of the dead at the end of time when, according to one view, body and soul are reunited, or according to the other view, persons are given new life as integrated wholes.

Health and disease

Christians hold a positive view of the *human body* and its natural environment. Genuine wellbeing from this perspective is not about fleeing the material world in favor of the spiritual. Neither is it a matter of escaping individuality in union with the Whole or Absolute. Rather, it is the balanced integration and successful functioning of all aspects of life: physical, mental, social, ethical, and spiritual.

At least *three types of disease* flow from this understanding of health. The first is the malady of partiality. This occurs when an individual or society wholly disregards some important aspect of life, such as sex or spirituality. A second type of disease is the malady of imbalance and disintegration. Succeeding financially but not in other areas of life is an example. A third type of disease is the malady of unsuccessful functioning. This is what many people think of when they hear the word "disease." An eye that does not see, an ear that does not hear, or a brain that does not think are signs of ill health. This is the type of disease that medical professionals can most easily and effectively address.

Christians look at *suffering* – prolonged or continuing pain of any sort – in three primary ways. Some believe that God determines exactly what happens in every case, right down to the smallest detail. For them all suffering is good because everything fits into God's overall plan. Other Christians recoil at this suggestion. For them suffering is not good even though God can often help those who suffer to transform it into something good. A third stance threads a path between the first two by distinguishing between existential (normal) and pathological (abnormal) types of suffering.

The suffering that parents often feel after all their children have moved away from home is an example of the first. Trying to escape *existential suffering* is not wise. Suffering from a malignancy is an example of the *pathological suffering*. According to this Christian stance, the second kind of suffering should be prevented or treated as aggressively as the first should be patiently endured.

When either pain or suffering is not outweighed by its offsetting benefits it is *evil*. Christians hold that this occurs in at least three ways. The first is *moral evil*. This is caused by the misuse of human freedom. Murdering a child is an obvious example. The second is *natural evil*, which occurs when something in the world of nature causes uncompensated pain or suffering. Tidal waves, earthquakes, and tornados are illustrations. The third, and by far the most difficult for many to contemplate, is *ecological evil*. This is the predatory nature of the whole of life, something most Christians see as a consequence of sin: nothing in this world lives without killing.

Many Christians acknowledge that the pervasiveness and apparent permanence of evil in its three forms is the single greatest challenge to Christian faith. This is because it is very difficult, both theoretically and experientially, to believe that the one true God is (1) wholly loving and (2) supremely powerful in light of (3) all the evil we observe and experience. This issue is often called the problem of *"theodicy,"* a Greek word made up of two others that mean "God" and "righteousness" or "justice."

Christians today relate to theodicy, or the problem of evil and suffering in the world as it relates to God, in three primary ways. Some come close to *denying that evil is real*. They say that life is like a movie and that once we have come to its end we will see that every scene was necessary. Or they say that life is more like a large painting. Its dark portions seem pointless when we stand too close. But when we stand back far enough to view it as a whole, we can see the contributions that even its shadows make.

Other Christians *qualify the idea that God is completely loving*. Some of these hold that even before they are conceived, God freely chooses whom he will love and whom he will hate. Others take a more measured approach. They contend that in our time the word "love" has become so sentimental that many take it for granted that it is better to feel good than to be good and to do good. Given this widespread meaning of the word "love," they contend that it is better not to apply it to God.

Yet other Christians take a hard look at the idea of *divine power*, recognizing that there are some things God cannot do. God cannot do that which is self-contradictory. For example, no matter how vigorous the effort, God cannot make 2 + 3 = 7. Also, God cannot do that which is contrary to God's own moral character. An example of this is that God cannot command the torture of innocent children or compel unfaithful spouses to stop cheating.

Taken together, these three *"limitations" on divine power* make it less plausible to hold God unilaterally responsible for evil. Yet even if this alternative reduces the perplexity and doubt that evil causes, something that many Christians doubt, it does not eliminate them. To some extent, this challenge to Christian faith always remains.

As Christians struggle to understand the meaning of pain and suffering on the macrocosmic level, they are also confronted with many health issues that demand decisions for moral and ethical living. Being in optimum health and making wise ethical decisions that impact one's health are not only a necessity for survival and vibrant living, but also a fulfilment of the divine mandate to be a caretaker of the gifts and resources granted by God.

All Christians take seriously Apostle Paul's words, "Whether you eat or drink or whatever you do, do it all for *the glory of God*" (1 Corinthians 10:31). We will see, however, that on some of the most talked-about and relevant health and bioethical issues of daily living, Christians are divided. In the paragraphs that follow, we survey five such issues – diet, procreation, abortion, stem cell research, and homosexuality.

For most Christians, the issue of *diet* is a very personal one. A great majority of Catholics, Protestants, and the Orthodox do not have imposed restrictions on diet – what one can consume and not. For them, the death of Jesus voided the distinction between clean and unclean meat that are found in the Old Testament and opened the avenue for a life of freedom on dietary matters as long as one's health is not injured.

A minority of Christians, however, hold that they have a religious duty to avoid food and substances that are known to have negative consequences. They have sometimes advocated vegetarianism as the ideal diet. Some hold that tobacco and alcohol have no place in a Christian's life.

This minority of Christians sometimes make abstaining from tobacco and alcoholic beverages, or sometimes even meat which the Bible calls "unclean," a requirement for full church membership.

Most Christians, however, do not follow such restrictions and argue instead that the freedom that Christians find in the salvation offered by Jesus allows them to make individual decisions on these matters. They would oppose excessive consumption of alcohol and meat, but do not find moral or biblical arguments against moderate consumption of either.

Historically, Christians have held strong views on *human sexuality*. Virtually all of them agree that this part of life has two purposes. One of these is the unitive purpose (making love) and the other is the procreative purpose (making babies). It is difficult to find Christians of any sort who object to this. Differences of conviction surface when it is asked whether it can be ethically permissible for husbands and wives intentionally to separate the two purposes.

Most Evangelical Protestants and Mainline Protestants agree that it is ethically acceptable to separate the unitive and procreative purposes. This is why they typically do not object to the judicious use of interventions such as contraception, artificial insemination, in vitro fertilization, and surrogate gestations.

Roman Catholicism teaches that it is not ethically permissible for husbands and wives intentionally to separate the unitive and procreative purposes. It opposes *sterilization, contraception, and abortion* partly because it believes that they violate the procreative purpose. It opposes *artificial insemination, in vitro fertilization, and surrogate gestation* partly because it believes that they violate the unitive purpose of sexual intimacy. It holds that each new human life should begin in love and that these technological interventions make this difficult or even impossible.

Christians differ sharply about *abortion* most of all. Mainline Protestants typically are willing to view it with regret but also with moral approval in cases like rape, incest, profound fetal malformation, and extreme maternal distress. They also agree that medical practice and public policies should enable each pregnant woman to decide for herself whether she will have an abortion.

Evangelicals, Roman Catholics, and Eastern Orthodox Christians oppose abortion unless it is required to save the pregnant woman's physical life and they favor outlawing it for any other reason.

The more comprehensive idea is that people should be seamlessly prolife from conception to the grave. This informs the Catholic position on *stem cell research* as well. The "when" question surfaces here as it does elsewhere. Those who hold that the new life should be protected from the time of conception onward necessarily oppose it. Those who believe that this should begin from the time of implantation or later can approve it. To be sure, however, all Christians place value on humankind from conception forward. It simply cannot be truthfully stated that Christians who allow for exceptions do so because they devalue human life in its nascent forms.

Homosexuality is another issue that divides Mainline Protestants, on the one hand, and Evangelical Protestants, Orthodox Christians, and Roman Catholics, on the other. Most in the second group view heterosexual identity as an aberration from God's created order and condemn homosexual practice as sinful. They believe that God's creation of Adam and Eve as heterosexuals is the norm.

Many in the Mainline Protestant churches hold that homosexuality is a trait as part of God's creative activity. They interpret the biblical condemnations of homosexual conduct as reflecting the cultural norms and biases of the time. Perhaps more clearly than anywhere else, on this issue we see the results of differing interpretive methods of reading scripture, viewing reality, and interacting with important ethical issues of our time.

With respect to homosexuality, the issue is complex. This is because on this one matter a significant number of Mainline Protestants agree with the Evangelicals and some Evangelicals agree with the Mainline Protestants. This is causing tensions and reconfigurations on both sides of the divide.

Death and dying

Virtually all Christians in the United States accept the two standard ways of understanding death. One of these is that death is the total and irreversible loss of circulatory (pulse) and respiratory (breath) functions. The other is that death is the irreversible loss of the functioning of the entire brain, including the stem. Though most Christians agree on the physiological meaning of death, the differences that lie among them on its theological meaning lead to different conclusions on such end-of-life bioethical issues as euthanasia and suicide.

The word "euthanasia" is an English term derived from the Greek language that literally means "good death," not "mercy killing." Deciding which kinds of death are genuinely good requires an individual or group to face two distinctions. One of these is the difference between voluntary euthanasia and non-voluntary euthanasia, the first being a death that a mentally competent patient chooses voluntarily and with adequate information.

Virtually all Christians approve of not always doing everything to keep a patient alive. They agree with the Bible that there is a time for everything, including a time to die, and that all others should respect this. About such measure – also called passive euthanasia – the consensus is overwhelming. However, most Christians – again most Roman Catholics, Evangelical Protestants, and Orthodox Christians – oppose active euthanasia which is intentionally and actively killing a patient.

A different situation is giving a terminally ill patient enough medicine to keep him or her comfortable even if doing this unintentionally causes him or her to die perhaps more swiftly. Making use of a longstanding distinction between foreseen and intended consequences, most Christians approve of this whether they are Roman Catholic, Mainline Protestants, or Evangelicals. As we see in a number of analogous cases, the distinction between foreseen and intended consequences can survive the reservations of those who doubt its usefulness.

One of these is that surgeons foresee that they will leave scars but do not intend to do so. Likewise, oncologists foresee that chemotherapy will have uncomfortable and unsightly side effects, but they do not intend this. Still further, those who apply radiation therapy foresee that they will probably damage some healthy flesh, but they do not intend this.

Such analogous situations can be identified almost endlessly. The way to know if an outcome is foreseen or intended is to see if any steps are being taken to mitigate it. If everything possible is being done to decrease negative outcomes, they are foreseen. If nothing along these lines is done, then we may conclude that they are either intended or the result of indifference, both of which are wholly unacceptable.

Suicide is seen with disapproval by most Christians, even though the biblical writers sometimes report that someone ended his or her own life without expressing moral approval or disapproval. Some have gone so far as to say that it is an "unpardonable sin" because it is the only one for which it is impossible to ask forgiveness. In previous generations, Christians have desecrated the bodies of those who committed suicide and denied them burial in Christian cemeteries. Few Christian groups approve of such treatment in the twenty-first century, almost all preferring to view one who has committed suicide as an individual who was overcome by difficulties in his or her life.

This negative attitude toward suicide is still evident in widespread Christian opposition to laws such as those that allow doctors to give patients prescriptions for lethal drugs with which they – the patients themselves, not the doctors – can end their own lives. Again, almost all Evangelical Protestants and Roman Catholics oppose it whereas a significant number of Mainline Protestants do not object to it.

Christians ritualize death and the grieving process in diverse ways but follow a common theme of hope and comfort. For Roman Catholics, it is important for the dying to receive the sacrament of prayer for the sick conducted by a priest in preparation for death. Once the patient dies, three rituals traditionally take place: (1) the vigil or wake at which family and friends spend prayerful time together with the deceased person; (2) a requiem mass at a church or cathedral which is led by a priest, and (3) the rite of committal where the loved one is laid to rest.

Protestants typically have three events that parallel these; however, they can be less formal and traditional. Protestants often hold separate meetings for: (1) the viewing of the deceased (now, only occasionally); (2) the funeral or memorial service led by a minister or a spiritual leader and involving family members; and (3) interment at the burial site.

Orthodox Christians have a four-part process: (1) the Trisagion service (to ask God to grant rest to the departed soul), which takes place the night before the funeral service at the wake; (2) the funeral service with an open casket at an Orthodox church led by a priest; (3) burial at graveside asking God again to give rest to the soul of the deceased; and (4) *Makaria*, a "mercy meal" shared by the mourners to celebrate the life of the deceased, traditionally with fish as a sign of fasting and mourning.

Christians are divided on the practice of cremation. Orthodoxy views cremation as desecration of the body, thus funeral services with cremated remains are not allowed in Orthodox churches. Until the 1960s, Roman Catholics were of the same position, but they have since relaxed their stance, allowing for individuals and families to decide and giving permission to priests to hold funeral masses with cremated remains. Evangelical and Mainline Protestants, on the other hand, leave the issue of the disposition of the body to the patients and their families.

Table 12.1 Dos and don'ts

Dos	Don'ts
1. Remember how large and diverse Christianity is.	1. Do not act as though all religious people are ignorant.
2. Keep in mind the general bioethical tendencies of Evangelical Protestants, Roman Catholics, and Mainline Protestants.	2. Do not think that if you know what one Christian believes you know what they all believe.
3. Understand the difference between foreseen and intended consequences and why many Christians think it matters.	3. Do not tell patients that suffering is part of God's plan.
4. Enlist the help of Christian chaplains, ministers, and priests.	4. Do not override the medical choices of mentally competent, informed, and un-coerced people because of your own religious beliefs.
5. Seek mentally competent, informed, and voluntary consent.	5. Do not assume that they will eat anything offered.
6. Relieve pain and suffering.	

Conclusion

Over the last 2,000 years, Christianity has made many twists and turns while never entirely losing its own identity. At this time in the United States, Christianity is a conglomerate of diverse theologies and historical expressions with Roman Catholics, Orthodox Christians, Evangelical Protestants, and Mainline Protestants aligning themselves in different ways from one issue to another. For the most part, although there are important exceptions, Catholics, Evangelical Protestants, and the Orthodox tend to represent the "conservative" wing of Christianity, while Mainline Protestants tend to occupy the "liberal" wing.

This pattern is evident and persistent in the relationships between these Christian groups and health and healing. Despite stark differences on a number of theological and bioethical issues, however, many Christians are still able to find connectedness with each other through their common commitment to understanding and applying the Bible, common faith in Jesus, and mutual engagement in the world for positive transformation.

Case study #1

The intake form indicated that the patient was a 37-year-old male who lived with his spouse and two children. The patient identified as a Pentecostal Christian and had recently moved from Florida to the Pacific Northwest. The patient shared that he had been experiencing low levels of energy and had been spending greater amounts of time in bed than usual. After an unremarkable medical work-up, his primary care provider referred him to a psychiatrist for treatment.

The psychiatrist reviewed the patient's intake form prior to their first session and diagnosed the patient with situational depression likely brought about by his relocation and separation from family in Florida. The psychiatrist recommended that the patient start an antidepressant to ease the adjustment with the hope that the depression would subside as he adjusted and acquainted himself with his new community.

The patient expressed concern around taking a pill every day to make his "problems go away." The patient shared that he relied on his "relationship with Jesus" to navigate his personal struggles and said: "Jesus is my antidepressant." He requested recommendations for non-pharmacological interventions to treat his depression.

Questions for reflection

1. Could an understanding of the patient's spiritual/religious values help the psychiatrist to better support him in his treatment? Why or why not?
2. How could the psychiatrist respectfully explore the patient's concerns around antidepressants? Why might the patient have some reservations about anti-depressants? How might his reservations relate to his religious beliefs?
3. The patient was seeking non-pharmacological interventions for depression while asserting that "Jesus is my antidepressant." Is this a contradiction? How might this make sense to the patient?
4. Pathways of communication with the unseen or the supernatural vary widely among religious persons. Would it be appropriate to inquire how the patient experiences his relationship with Jesus?

*Submitted by Garrett Potts

Case study #2

A 15-year-old female came to her dermatologist seeking treatment for severe acne. The patient's mother joined her for the appointment. Both the patient and her mother were Roman Catholic and expressed that their values were informed by their Catholic faith. After he reviewed some bloodwork, the dermatologist determined that the patient would be a good candidate for *Accutane*, a brand-named version of Isotretinoin used when other acne treatments have not been successful.

The doctor explained to the patient and her mother that the government mandates that any female prescribed *Accutane* must take a pregnancy test and be on two forms of birth control. This regulation is necessary because the medication has been known to cause serious birth defects. Without meeting these requirements, providers are unable to prescribe the drug.

The patient's mother expressed a strong moral conviction against the idea of her daughter taking birth control. The patient pleaded with her mother to allow her to take the medication, having been very self-conscious about her acne. The patient's mother said that she trusted that her daughter would remain abstinent if prescribed birth control, but she disagreed with the idea of her daughter being on birth control on principle.

Two weeks later, this provider cared for another Catholic teenage female accompanied by her mother who expressed no concern about her daughter being on birth control.

Questions for reflection

1. How can the patient's and her mother's values be explained by their Catholic beliefs? Discuss potential differences in their respective orientations to their belief system.
2. How would you support the family's spiritual/religious values and medical needs if you were their provider?

3. Was it appropriate for the dermatologist to recommend *Accutane* as a possible treatment for a Catholic? Is it reasonable to assume his coursework in pharmacology included this information?

Submitted by Garrett Potts

Glossary

Body of Christ Either the Christian church as the continuation of the ministry of Jesus Christ or the substance of the bread after it has been changed into the body of Jesus Christ in the Mass.

Deism Reduction of religion to what reason can establish; belief that God created the world but that now it functions on its own; partly a religious response to the European Enlightenment.

Eastern Orthodoxy One of the three major branches of Christianity first centered in the Eastern portion of the Roman Empire but now worldwide; originally Greek in language and culture.

Evangelical Awakening Widespread and somewhat emotional revival in eighteenth-century England and North America of Christianity; partly a religious response to the European Enlightenment.

Fundamentalism Intensely negative reactions among twentieth-century Protestants primarily in North America against attempts to modernize Christianity; sought to get "back to basics."

Protestantism, Evangelical More conservative Christian churches in the United States that descend from the sixteenth-century revolts against Roman Catholicism led by Martin Luther and others. Simply "Protestant" in much of Europe.

Protestant, Historically Black African American Christian churches in the United States that descend theologically from the sixteenth-century revolts against Roman Catholicism led by Martin Luther and others.

Protestantism, Mainline More liberal Christian churches in the United States that descend from the sixteenth-century revolts against Roman Catholicism led by Martin Luther and others.

Roman Catholicism One of the three major branches of Christianity first centered in the Western portion of the Roman Empire but now worldwide; originally Latin in language and culture.

Sacrament Christian ritual or practice that conveys divine grace in human life. A "visible sign of an invisible reality."

Sin Thought, word, or deed contrary to the will of God. "Original sin" used as a theological term refers to the first sin by the first humans, Adam and Eve. The subsequent negative consequences of this original sin affect the lives of each human person.

Trinity The only true God, who exists of one substance in three persons, in whom Christians believe.

Note

1 All scripture references utilize the *New Revised Standard Version Bible (Anglicized) With Aprocrypha* (1995).

Bibliography

American Demografia (2022) "Religion in the United States, 2022." https://uscanadainfo.com/religion-in-the-united-states/

Chalcedon Creed (451 ce) *Center for Reformed Theology and Apologetics*. www.apuritansmind.com/creeds-and-confessions/the-chalcedonian-creed-circa-451-a-d/

Edwards, J. (1959) *Religious Affections: The Works of Jonathan Edwards*, vol. 2, Smith, JE. (ed.) New Haven: Yale University Press.

Great Disappointment (2023, March 23) *Wikipedia*. https://en.wikipedia.org/wiki/Great_Disappointment.

New Revised Standard Version Bible (Anglicized) With Apocrypha (1995) New York: Oxford University Press.

Nicene Creed (325 ce) Center for Reformed Theology and Apologetics. www.apuritansmind.com/creeds-and-confessions/nicene-creed/

Pew Research Center (2012) "The Global Religious Landscape." www.pewresearch.org/religion/2012/12/18/global-religious-landscape-exec/

Pew Research Center (2017) "The Changing Global Religious Landscape." www.pewresearch.org/religion/2017/04/05/the-changing-global-religious-landscape/

Pew Research Center (2022) "Modeling the Future of Religion in America." www.pewresearch.org/religion/2022/09/13/how-u-s-religious-composition-has-changed-in-recent-decades/

Public Religion Research Institute (2021) "The 2020 Census of American Religion." www.prri.org/research/2020-census-of-american-religion/

Statista (2021) "Self-Described Religious Identification in the Adult Population in the United States, 2021." www.statista.com/statistics/183817/religious-identification-of-adult-population/

13 Four distinctive Christian denominations

Julius J. Nam[1]

All who have died without a knowledge of this gospel, who would have received it if they had been permitted to tarry, shall be heirs of the celestial kingdom of God. Also all that shall die henceforth without a knowledge of it, who would have received it with all their hearts, shall be heirs of that kingdom. For I, the Lord, will judge all men according to their works, according to the desire of their hearts.

(Joseph Smith. Jr. n.d.)

As the health of invalids improves under judicious treatment, and they begin to enjoy life, they have confidence in those who have been instrumental in their restoration to health. Their hearts are filled with gratitude, and the good seed of truth will the more readily find a lodgement there and in some cases will be nourished, spring up, and bear fruit to the glory of God. One such precious soul saved will be worth more than all the means needed to establish such an institution.

(Ellen G. White, 1914)

There is no life, truth, intelligence, nor substance in matter. All is infinite Mind and its infinite manifestation, for God is All-in-all. Spirit is immortal Truth; matter is mortal error. Spirit is the real and eternal; matter is the unreal and temporal. Spirit is God, and man is His image and likeness. Therefore, man is not material; he is spiritual.

(Mary Baker Eddy, 1907)

The world is fast coming to realize that the "kingdoms of this world" are not Christlike, and that their claim to be of Christ's appointment is not unquestionable. Men are beginning to use their reasoning powers on this and similar questions; and they will act out their convictions so much more violently, as they come to realize that a deception has been practiced upon them in the name of the God of Justice and the Prince of Peace. In fact, the tendency with many is to conclude that Christianity itself is an imposition without foundation, and that, leagued with civil rulers, its aim is merely to hold in check the liberties of the masses.

(Charles Taze Russell, 1886)

Introduction

America, in the mid-nineteenth century, was a place of great religious ferment. The Second Great Awakening of the 1820s and 1830s brought a new revival in personal religion and spirituality among Protestant Christians. Protestants, who comprised the dominant majority, continued to carry the belief that America was a land of destiny with a special purpose in the world. This belief, as well as a sense of optimism and adventure

DOI: 10.4324/9781003288862-13

that came with the founding of the new nation and the modern progress in science, technology, and industry, contributed to the flowering of new religious and social movements that sought reform in religion and society.

Each of the religious movements discussed in this chapter arose as an expression of and response to that reform impulse in nineteenth-century America. Each presented a strong, unique vision of religion and American society and demanded radical dedication to the faith and practice of the community. Each became a denomination.

While Latter-day Saints, Seventh-day Adventists, Christian Scientists, and Jehovah's Witnesses all base their beliefs on the Bible and confess Jesus Christ as their Lord much like most other Christians, they have distinct beliefs and practices on health that set them apart. Still, all four of these groups share the general Christian commitment to physical, emotional, and relational health, based on the biblical teaching that the human body is a "temple of the Holy Spirit" (*New Revised Standard Version Bible* 1995: 1 Corinthians 6:19). It is on the specific interpretation and application of the Bible's teachings on health that they differ.

Latter-day Saints

Demographics

As of 2022, the Church of Jesus Christ of Latter-day Saints reported worldwide membership of 16.8 million in more than 31,000 wards (equivalent to local congregations). The United States had the highest number with 6.7 million. Within the US, the western states of Utah, California, Idaho, and Arizona had the highest number – with Utah leading the way with two million. Globally, the church was active in more than 120 countries, especially in Central and South American countries, Australia, Canada, Japan, the Philippines, and the United Kingdom. Mexico and Brazil had the largest number of Latter-day Saints outside of the United States, each with about 1.4 million (Church of Jesus Christ of Latter-day Saints 2022).

History

The Church of Jesus Christ of Latter-day Saints (or Mormonism as it is popularly called) was established in April 1830 in New York by Joseph Smith (1805–1844). Smith claimed to have received visions from God who instructed him to restore the true church of Christ. An angel named Moroni directed Smith to long-hidden golden plates containing stories of God's people in the North American continent going back to 600 BCE, Jesus' revelations to Native Americans in the first century CE, and subsequent experiences of Christians in America. These golden plates were translated into English and took the name of the *Book of Mormon*. As a record of the direct revelation of Jesus, the *Book of Mormon* was considered to be of equal authority to the Bible. The restoration of the true church included acceptance of the *Book of Mormon* and Joseph Smith as a modern-day prophet.

The distinct claims of Latter-day Saints resulted in persecution of the group by Protestants, which compelled the movement to become an itinerant community. Between 1830 and 1844, Latter-day Saints moved from New York to Ohio to Missouri to Illinois, where an anti-Mormon mob killed Smith and his brother. This led them far west beyond the then-borders of the United States to what is now Utah under the leadership of Brigham Young (1801–1877), the church's second prophet – one of the tenets of the Latter-day Saint belief system being the continuing gift of prophecy in modern times. Young guided the church through the difficult early years in Utah and toward becoming the thriving global movement that it is today.

Beliefs

As the full name of their church indicates, Latter-day Saints clearly view their movement as a Christian church. However, they see themselves as belonging to neither the Catholic, the Orthodox, nor the Protestant tradition. Rather, they present their community as an independent branch that was raised up by God as the restoration of the true church instituted by Jesus Christ in the first century CE.

At the heart of that restoration lie their distinctive teachings on scripture, the Godhead, and the church. Latter-day Saints affirm scripture as recognized by Protestants (predominantly, the King James Version). But they differ from both Protestants and Catholics in that they accept additional writings as part of the scriptural canon: *The Book of Mormon* (believed to be a revelation of Jesus Christ given to Native Americans), *Pearl of Great Price* (Joseph Smith's corrections to the King James Version and translation of other documents), and *Doctrine and Covenants* (the prophecies of Joseph Smith and all his successors down to the present). The recognition of the latter book is based on the Latter-day Saint teaching that the gift of prophecy (and the inspired authority that comes with it) continues in the present age through the prophet of the church who serves also as the president.

Another key difference between Latter-day Saints and other Christians is on the understanding of the Godhead. Latter-day Saints view God the Father, his Son (Jesus Christ), and the Holy Spirit as three distinct persons. They understand Jesus to be a literal and physical son of God the Father – thus, subservient in authority to the Father. Still, like other Christian movements, they do believe in the incarnation of Jesus – that he left the spiritual realms to become a human being in flesh – and in salvation of humankind through faith in Jesus. Finally, the Latter-day Saint conviction that their movement is the restoration of the true church of Jesus Christ at the end of earth's history (hence, "Latter-day" Saints) leads them to hold that the ordinances of their church have unique efficacy in the world that is to come. They believe that to reach the highest degree of salvation, or exaltation, one must participate in the "saving ordinances" of their church, including particular washings, anointing, and celestial marriage, which, on earth, is available only in the church's temple.

Health and disease

Latter-day Saints, Seventh-day Adventists, and Jehovah's Witnesses view diseases and illnesses as consequences of sin. Based upon passages in the Old Testament, they view sin as having entered the universe through archangel Lucifer's rebellion against God. After his rebellion, Lucifer is also known as Satan or the Devil, who tempted and deceived Adam and Eve, the first human beings created by God and placed in the paradisiacal Garden of Eden. Adam and Eve were indeed deceived and their "fall" is how sin entered the world. Sin is defined as disobedience and rebellion against God and it has resulted in pain, suffering, further disobedience, broken relationships and environment, and ultimately death.

The three traditions commonly hold that sin has created physical and environmental conditions leading to physical and psychological dysfunctions, diseases, and illnesses. They also hold that the intemperate choices that individuals make – which are also consequences of the sinful condition of the world – contribute to sickness of all types. They do not distinguish between physical and mental illnesses, but view both in physical and spiritual terms. These illnesses have natural, physiological causes that can be managed or overcome through modern medicine.

Latter-day Saints believe that it is a religious duty to take good care of the physical body with which the spirit is united during life on earth. The body is considered a gift from God which plays an important part in one's "eternal progression," the process of growth toward perfection that began before birth and will continue forever. What happens to the body and how one takes care of the body have consequences that go beyond this life. They also teach that the family is the basic unit of the church and the basis for a righteous, holy life. Every person is viewed as a child of heavenly as well as human parents, as each in his or her premortal life was created by the Heavenly Father and Heavenly Mother and part of the eternal family. Through birth, the person who was in the spirit state is joined with a physical body so that one can go through the process of eternal progression and reach higher levels in the spiritual realms.

Based on this belief, devout Latter-day Saints consider consumption of alcohol, tobacco, coffee, tea, and narcotics as violations of God's health laws. Coffee and tea are not to be taken due to their caffeine content, which can be habit-forming. Latter-day Saints tend to avoid other caffeinated drinks, such as cola products, as they too can be habit-forming, though technically this latter injunction is not considered to be mandatory. As for the dietary concerns, Latter-day Saints believe that all will become vegetarians during the Millennium, the 1,000-year period of peace which will commence with the second coming of Jesus, but none are required to be vegetarians. Still, meat is to be eaten sparingly, and all are encouraged to consume vegetables, fruits, and grains. These teachings are based on "Word of Wisdom," a section of *Doctrine and Covenants*, the 1835 book by Joseph Smith, which is considered part of scripture by Latter-day Saints.

On a number of sexual and biomedical issues, Latter-day Saints hold conservative positions. They believe that sexual activity, including passionate kissing, outside of marriage is wrong. Although until 1890 they believed in and practiced polygamy, they teach monogamy – union of a man and a woman – as the only norm for marriage. They consider homosexuality a sinful condition and condemn its practice as unbiblical and unnatural. They oppose abortion, considering it a violation of the commandment not to kill (*New Revised Standard Version Bible* 1995: Exodus 20:13). Only in extraordinary circumstances can abortion be permitted – in cases of rape, incest, grave danger to the mother's life or health, and fatal defect in the fetus. In such situations, they are instructed to consult church leaders and give time for prayerful consideration before deciding on abortion. Latter-day Saints do not approve of artificial insemination except within a marriage relationship. They also discourage using genetic materials other than the husband's or the wife's. At the same time, this decision is ultimately left up to the couple. On the issue of birth control, Latter-day Saints do not have a mandatory rule for all. However, because of the importance they place on family and the responsibility to bear children, they have historically encouraged child bearing and discouraged permanent birth control methods such as vasectomies, tied fallopian tubes, and premature hysterec-tomies. But, in the end, the decision remains with the couple.

Death

Latter-day Saints' belief in life after death allows them to accept it as the passage to the next phase of life, though they neither seek it nor embrace it openly. Upon death, all will proceed to the spirit world until the day of Jesus' second coming and resurrection of these spirits. At that time, all will be assigned to different levels of God's kingdom according to their actions and affiliations while on earth. Opportunities for accepting Jesus will be given to spirits even at that time and those who do accept him will join the process of "eternal progression" toward the status of divinity. Satan, his devils, and those who per-sist in rebellion against God will be thrown into "outer darkness" as eternal punishment.

Latter-day Saints are encouraged to bury their dead in the ground in keeping with the biblical practice of returning "dust to dust." However, if the local law requires, other practices such as cremation are allowed. Latter-day Saints who have received the "Temple Endowment," a particular privilege to take part in temple services, are dressed in a temple garment before burial – with the women of the Relief Society dressing women and men who have been ordained as priests dressing men. Typically, a funeral and/or graveside service presided by a bishop or his representative precedes the burial. The burial may include the dedication of the grave as a holy resting place until the day of resurrection. The grave then becomes a sacred site for the family of the deceased. Suicide is denounced as wrong, but Latter-day Saints reserve the ultimate judgment to God. They generally condemn physician-assisted suicide and active euthanasia, but give room for allowing patients to pass away rather than keeping them alive in vegetative or extremely painful and miserable conditions in the final stages of terminal illnesses. In such dire situations, the decision is left to the patients and their families and caregivers. Autopsies may be performed, if required by law and/or consented by the family of the deceased.

Seventh-day Adventism

Demographics

As of 2021, the Seventh-day Adventist Church had 21.9 million members worldwide in 92,876 local churches. Adventists have an active church presence in 212 nations (Seventh-day Adventist Church 2021). India had the highest number of Adventists in any country with 1.5 million, with Brazil coming a close second with 1.45 million. In 2015, the United States had just over one million with California having the highest number of Adventist residents (Seventh-day Adventist Church 2015). Church membership was particularly strong in eastern and southern Africa, the American continents, parts of Southeast Asia, and the Indian sub-continent. With the financial support of many indi-viduals and organizations, its *Adventist Development and Relief Services Agency* serves 22 million people in 18 nations per year (Seventh-day Adventist Church 2015).

History

The year of Joseph Smith's death, 1844, is significant for Seventh-day Adventists for a different reason. That was the predicted year of Jesus' second coming for the followers of

William Miller (1782–1849). Miller interpreted the 2,300-day prophecy of Daniel 8 as pointing to the return of Jesus and the end of history on October 22, 1844. Out of what came to be known as the Great Disappointment experience of that day, a group arose who reinterpreted the prophecy in Daniel 8 as referring to the *beginning* of the final phase in earth's history and adopted the seventh-day Sabbath as the true day of worship and the end-time sign of faithfulness to God. This group, eventually known as Seventh-day Adventists, was led by James White (1821–1881) and his wife, Ellen White (1827–1915), who from 1844 claimed to receive visions from God.

In the 1840s and 1850s, Adventists' preoccupation with Christ's imminent return prevented them from engaging in active missionary work or building institutions. However, by 1863, as the church grew, Adventists organized the church formally, with their headquarters located in Battle Creek, Michigan. The formal organization of the church launched Adventists on the path of building significant publishing, educational, and medical institutions through the United States and eventually the world as they aggressively embraced missionary outreach. Significant in this process was the work of Ellen White, who shaped Adventist thought and practice through her writings on the Bible, theology, lifestyle, church work, and mission.

Beliefs

Unlike Latter-day Saints, Adventists view themselves as belonging to the family of Protestant churches and adhere to the great Reformation principles of the supreme authority of the Bible, salvation by grace and faith in Jesus Christ, and the priesthood of all believers (the idea that each believer can approach God directly and that each has a divine calling to minister to the world). They also agree with the historic Christian teachings on the Trinity, the divine-human nature of Jesus, and the importance of the church community as a manifestation of the invisible "Body of Christ."

At the same time, they hold some beliefs that distinguish them from other Protestant bodies. Among them are the teachings on Jesus' work in the heavenly sanctuary and the end-time, the Sabbath, and the gift of prophecy. When the Millerite expectation of Jesus' second coming on October 22, 1844, ended in what has come to be known as the Great Disappointment, a small group of would-be Seventh-day Adventists banded together to introduce a new interpretation claiming that Jesus, instead of returning to the earth, entered the Most Holy Place (the divine throne room) of the heavenly temple. This, they believed, was the beginning of the final period in earth's history during which Jesus was engaged in the investigation of all of humanity – dead and alive – to vindicate the true character of God and make the final determination of those eligible for eternal life. Since then, this belief has gone through several refinements, but Adventists remain officially committed to the belief that the final period in earth's history began in 1844 and that Jesus is engaged in a special end-time work in heaven. While this "sanctuary doctrine" was being developed, another of Adventism's distinctives was also being formulated – the recovery of the seventh-day Sabbath. Early Adventists believed that the "Christian Sabbath" of Sunday represented departure from the biblical Sabbath of both the Old and the New Testaments, which, they preached, was the same as the seventh-day Sabbath of the Jews. They further taught – and Adventists continue to teach – that the keeping of the Sabbath has special significance as a test of loyalty in the final days of earth's history. Finally, like Latter-day Saints, Adventists believe that the biblical gift of prophecy has continued throughout Christian history and was given to Ellen White, one of the founders of the church. Though she never claimed to be a "prophet" and the acceptance of her writings is not a condition for membership in the Adventist church, White is widely considered to have received the prophetic gift and her writings, though subservient in authority to scripture, hold a special value in the life of the community.

Health and disease

"The health message," as referred to by Seventh-day Adventists, is a major component of their beliefs and practices. This teaching began to develop soon after the church's formal organization in 1863 after Ellen White claimed to receive a vision about the importance of physical health and its connection to the mind and spirit. In 1865, White reported another vision in which she was given the message to start a medical institution. This resulted in the first Adventist healthcare institution, the first of hundreds to follow.

Helped by White, Adventists soon made the link between their health teachings and their belief about the human nature. Unlike most other Christians, Adventists hold that human beings are indivisible, organic unions of the body, mind, and spirit. Rejecting the view that human nature is composed of the body and the soul, they believe that the human person is the soul who completely ceases to exist at the time of death (without the "soul" going to heaven or hell). Because they view human nature as a composite of the body, mind, and spirit, they have found a deeper reason to value wholeness – harmonious development of the physical, mental, and spiritual health – even claiming that this experience of wholeness is part of one's preparation for the second coming of Christ.

In practical terms, the Adventist emphasis on health has led the church to promote healthy diet and lifestyle. Adventists condemn the use of alcohol, tobacco, and narcotics and recommend against caffeinated drinks such as coffee and tea. They teach vegetarianism as the recommended dietary norm and refrain from unclean meat as described in the Old Testament book Leviticus, chapter 11. There, "unclean meat" is the meat of animals that do not have split hoofs or chew the cud and the fish and seafood that do not have fins and scales. At the same time, dietary decisions are ultimately left up to the individual. Adventists are active in smoking-cessation efforts, prevention and treatment of alcohol use, and promotion of vegetarianism through their global network of healthcare institutions.

Like Latter-day Saints, Adventists tend to lean toward the conservative side of the social spectrum on issues dealing with sexuality and biomedical ethics. Adventists do not condone premarital or extramarital sexual activity, though the extent to which one engages in expressions of affection prior to intercourse is left up to the individual. Because they hold that appropriate sexual intimacy can occur only between a man and a woman in a marital relationship, Adventists do not accept homosexual romantic relationships or practices as legitimate. Abortion is unacceptable when it is performed as a means of birth control. Understanding it to be tragic, there are occasions, such as rape and/or incest, when abortion is thought to be justifiable. Adventists leave the final decision to the woman. Decisions on birth control and various methods of assisted human reproduction, including artificial insemination, are left up to the individuals involved.

Death

While Seventh-day Adventists view death as an abhorrent consequence of sin, they emphasize the hope that they hold for resurrection at the time of Jesus' second coming.

As noted already, Adventists believe that one goes neither to heaven nor hell after death, but the soul (i.e., the person) dies and ceases to exist. Their hope lies completely in God's power and promise of resurrection. The wicked, who persist in rebellion against God until the time of death, are expected to receive the final judgment of complete non-existence, which constitutes the Adventist understanding of hell. While they believe heaven to be a literal place, Adventists do not believe that hell represents an actual location but a metaphor for eternal non-existence.

Adventists do not have a prescribed ritual connected with death, though they typically hold funeral and burial services to celebrate the life of the deceased and encourage the loved ones in the knowledge that she/he rests in peaceful sleep until the coming of the Lord. These services are similar to most Protestant funeral rites; they involve singing of hymns, reading of scripture, pastoral homilies, tributes by family and friends, and prayers. Both burial and cremation are acceptable, and autopsies may be performed. While efforts to prolong life are positively viewed by Adventists, they do not oppose cessation of life support when signs of consciousness and of the possibility for recovery have ceased. They oppose suicide, assisted suicide, and active euthanasia, though the church's response in such difficult situations is one of ministry and support, rather than condemnation.

Christian Science

Demographics

Per instructions by Mary Baker Eddy, the founder of the Church of Christ, Scientist, Christian Scientists do not publish actual membership figures. Estimates vary greatly from 100,000 to 400,000 globally in 130 countries with more than 2,000 churches. Groups affiliated with the Church of Christ, Scientist, such as reading rooms, publishers, and social service enterprises as well as churches, are active in 80 countries. The churches are called branches of the "Mother Church" in Boston, Massachusetts. As of 2022, there were over 780 certified Christian Science practitioners (healers) listed in the directory *Christian Science Journal*, a monthly publication owned by the church (The Christian Science Journal 2022).

History

The Church of Christ, Scientist, was officially organized in 1879 in Lynn, Massachusetts, by Mary Baker Eddy (1821–1910). Like Joseph Smith and Ellen White, Eddy claimed to have a special experience with God and taught a distinct set of beliefs that stood in clear contrast with the dominant New England Protestantism of her time. Eddy, who grew up as a Congregationalist Christian, is said to have "discovered" Christian Science through a miraculous healing she experienced after a bad fall on the ice in February 1866. Initially, due to the severity of the fall, Eddy was thought to be dying. But after just three days of Bible reading while confined to bed, she made a dramatic recovery and "discovered" the true science of healing, particularly after her reading of Jesus' healing of a "palsied man" in Mark 9. This science, she believed, was to recognize that all reality is spiritual and to rely completely on life in the Spirit (see section "Beliefs and practices" for further clarification).

Eddy's teachings are captured in her 1875 book, which she expanded in 1883, with biblical expositions under the title *Science and Health with Key to the Scriptures*. Christian Scientists consider this book to be an inspired writing in addition to the Bible. In 1881, Eddy founded the Massachusetts Metaphysical College through which she spread her teachings on spirituality and healing. The following year, three years after the church was formally organized, the church headquarters moved from Lynn to Boston, signaling a more public phase of the community's outreach and growth. Though the teachings of Christian Science were directly at odds with the prevailing notions of knowledge, medicine, and religion, the very distinctive beliefs gave Christian Scientists a stronger and sharper identity and aided the community's international outreach.

Beliefs

Like Latter-day Saints, Christian Science does not see itself as belonging to any of the historic streams of Christianity. Rather, it claims to be a separate, unique phenomenon that recovers the healing power of God and the truth about reality. They agree with other Christians that the Bible is God's revelation and that Jesus who was the divine son of God was born of virgin birth and was resurrected after being crucified. They, however, do not read the Bible literally, but primarily metaphorically and allegorically, resulting in a theological system very different from most other Christian bodies.

Apart from their views on sin, death, metaphysics, and healing, which are discussed later in this chapter, other areas of uniqueness for Christian Science include their views on God the Father and Jesus Christ. Christian Scientists used the term "Trinity" to refer to the three-person Godhead of the Father, Christ, and the Holy Spirit, but their conception of the three is unique. For them, God is both a father and a mother figure who is different from Christ, the spiritual manifestation of God. God is simultaneously identifiable as the distinct "Divine Mind" and all of reality. Christ, then, is a manifestation of God which came to physical reality and became Jesus the human. Jesus was able to heal and perform other miracles because of Christ's manifestation of God in and through him. However, Christian Science distinguishes Jesus from Christ, teaching that the former was merely the bodily existence displaying Christ. Through this Jesus, though, God pointed to the true nature of reality – that it is spiritual – and the power available to all human beings from God through prayer.

Health and disease

Christian Scientists do not locate the cause of human suffering in one historical event, whether it is Lucifer's rebellion or the fall of Adam and Eve. In fact, they do not take the biblical story of creation and fall as historical accounts. They only take the story of Adam and Eve as allegories that teach the nature of sin, which they define as fear and ignorance. Diseases and illnesses, according to Christian Scientists, are the result of human ignorance about the true nature of God, or the Divine Mind, and reality. They teach that God loves every individual and that true reality is spiritual and non-material. They assert that the physicality and sickness as typically experienced by human beings are illusory. Once individuals abandon false understandings of God and reality and experience re-orientation of thought toward the true reality that is spiritual, sickness will disappear, even in this life. As noted already, due to such a strong belief in the spiritual nature of healing, Christian Scientists generally avoid modern medical care, including blood transfusion, organ transplantation, and drugs that affect the mind, such as pain medication.

Death

Death for Christian Scientists is an illusion. It, along with decay and sickness in life, is a result of erroneous understanding of God and the spiritual nature of reality. Thus, with proper understanding and insight, it can be overcome. When one does die, Christian Scientists do not consider the event as necessarily a tragedy as it represents release into the mental, spiritual state of existence where the individual's consciousness will continue in its quest for purer understanding of God and reality. Christian Scientists believe that this process of "purification" will continue forever with neither reward nor punishment awaiting the end of this life or future transitions in phases of existence.

Christian Scientists do not have a pre-determined method of marking death or preparing for death. Given their particular view toward modern medicine, it would be important to ascertain the exact wishes of the patients and their families nearing death as to how they wish to receive medical care, if at all. The church does not have an official position on euthanasia or assisted suicide, though suicide in general is considered to be against the divine principle of life. All decisions – including the method of disposition of the body – are left to the dying and their families. Christian Scientists hold memorial services typically at home or the funeral home. Since they do not have ordained clergy, family members or recognized leaders of the local Christian Science community may preside.

Jehovah's Witnesses

Demographics

As of 2022, almost nine million Jehovah's Witnesses reported worshiping worldwide every week in about 118,000 congregations in 239 countries (Jehovah's Witnesses 2022). The United States has the highest number of Witnesses with 1.2 million, with Mexico and Brazil tying for second place around 800,000. As with many other Christian movements, their numbers are particularly strong in Central and South American countries and Eastern Europe. Within the United States, higher concentrations of Jehovah's Witnesses are found in southern and western states. They are most famous for their 8.7 million evangelists who walk door to door distributing their journals *Watch Tower* and *Awake* and conversing with people about their beliefs whenever they can (Jehovah's Witnesses 2014).

History

The Jehovah's Witnesses were the last of these four groups to appear on the American religious landscape. After being involved in failed date-setting efforts for the second coming of Jesus Christ, Presbyterian-turned-Congregationalist Charles Taze Russell (1852–1916) formed his own apocalyptic Christian movement in 1879, whose primary activity was the publication of *Zion's Watch Tower and Herald of Christ's Presence*. Through this periodical, Russell advanced his own interpretation of the end-time prophecies of scripture, which included the belief that Christ had already come invisibly and his presence was increasingly being manifested in the world. Within a year, more than 30 groups formed in connection with *Zion's Watch Tower*, leading to the incorporation of the Watch Tower Bible and Tract Society in 1884. Though Russell never claimed inspiration or prophetic calling, his interpretations of scripture, including his belief that Christ's presence would reach its peak in 1914 and that World War I was the biblical Battle of Armageddon, was normative for all the members of the Watch Tower Society.

After Russell died in 1916, Joseph F. Rutherford (1869–1942) succeeded Russell as the Society's second president. It was under Rutherford's leadership that the society began calling itself Jehovah's Witnesses in 1931. Rutherford made some revisions to Russell's interpretations, including the identification of Armageddon with World War I, and added some new predictions, including the failed claim that Old Testament patriarchs would be resurrected beginning in 1925. Another of Rutherford's innovations was resistance to governmental authority. He taught the Witnesses to resist military service and all political activity. Although the Witnesses have since experienced further failures of prophecies by their leaders and persecution from states that have not respected their conscientious objection stance toward military service, they have persevered and grown stronger through aggressive evangelistic outreach both within the US and throughout the world.

Beliefs and practices

As part of their commitment to the body as the temple of the Holy Spirit, Jehovah's Witnesses value healthful living in all areas of life. As with Seventh-day Adventists, Jehovah's Witnesses hold the view that the human soul is mortal and integrated with the body. Thus, they believe that the soul dies at the time of death and becomes nothing – until the time of the second coming of Jesus, who will resurrect the saints to eternal life. But, unlike Seventh-day Adventists, Jehovah's Witnesses have not made this belief an essential part of their mission and global health work.

One key distinctive mark of Jehovah's Witnesses' teachings about health focuses on human blood. They take literally such biblical passages as Leviticus 17:10, 11, where God condemns eating of meat that has not had the blood removed (kosher meat) and Acts 15:28 where Christians are instructed to abstain from blood. This is so because blood, according to the Bible, represents life. Acceptance of these passages has led Witnesses to rule out consumption, storage, and transfusion of blood or any of its parts at all times – even when threatened by death. They are also discouraged from receiving organ transplantation since others' blood may be introduced to their bodies through the organs. This belief regarding blood has stimulated Witnesses to seek alternatives to medical procedures that involve blood transfusions, leading to innovations in bloodless surgery techniques. The church's Hospital Information Services promotes greater public awareness of bloodless surgery and facilitates such procedures for its members with cooperative medical institutions.

Though Jehovah's Witnesses notably take exception to the transfusion and storage of blood, they do not see utilization of modern medicine and naturalistic scientific understanding and practices as running counter to their belief in the spiritual dimension of human suffering. Prayer for healing does accompany the employment of modern healthcare, though individuals in each of the three traditions recognize that ultimate healing will only be possible when the fundamental cause of sickness – the sinful, corrupted condition of the world – is overcome at the time of the second coming of Jesus. At that time, Jesus will eradicate sin from the earth and bring about a perfect, sinless, disease-free state of being.

Death

Jehovah's Witnesses view death, hell, and the nature of afterlife in the same way as Seventh-day Adventists. They also believe that death and hell mean complete non-existence and that the righteous will be resurrected (i.e., given new existence) at the time of Jesus' second coming and live forever with God experiencing the reward of eternal life.

Care for the dying and disposition of the dead are largely left to the individuals and their families. While they do not believe that scripture requires indefinite life support, Jehovah's Witnesses believe in maximizing the length and quality of life. Thus, they oppose suicide, assisted suicide, and active euthanasia. Autopsies of the deceased are accepted, as are cremation and burial, depending on the wishes of the families. No particular funeral services are prescribed for Jehovah's Witnesses, though typically a "memorial talk" will be held at the Witnesses' Kingdom Hall or a funeral home, followed by a graveside service. These services consist of a homily by a community leader based on scripture and prayers of comfort for the families.

As with the other three groups, Jehovah's Witnesses hold conservative views on sexuality and many lifestyle issues. They view marriage as taking place only between a man and a woman and condemn premarital and extramarital sex and homosexuality as sinful. They also condemn abortion and assisted reproductive measures that involve semen or eggs of individuals other than the couple involved. As for dietary concerns, Jehovah's Witnesses do not have particular restrictions, except for consumption of meat with blood in it. They abstain from certain substances such as tobacco and narcotics, but alcoholic and caffeinated beverages are acceptable as long as individuals consume them in moderation.

Summary

Though Latter-day Saints, Seventh-day Adventists, Christian Scientists, and Jehovah's Witnesses share many important commonalities with other Christian traditions, such as Catholicism and mainline and evangelical Protestant groups, they bear some prominent beliefs and practices on health, human nature, and death that set them apart. The distinguishing features result from each group's different interpretations of scripture's teachings on health, sin, human nature, and reality, though the four do share a generally similar outlook on sexual morality and importance of right, healthful living.

Each in its own way represents a response to the challenges that the advancement of modern medicine posed to nineteenth-century America. Latter-day Saints and Seventh-day Adventists showed great openness to the healing methods of modern medicine and allowed the best of science to inform their health practices. Jehovah's Witnesses generally followed the same path, though they could not embrace modern medicine as openly as the former two due to the literal reading of scripture's teachings on blood. On the other hand, Christian Science represents the strongest exception taken to modern medicine, denying its premise of viewing reality as material.

The Christian Scientist rejection of all modern medicine in favor of its own methods of healing, and the narrower Jehovah's Witness rejection of most types of blood transfusions, frequently create ethical and legal questions in clinical settings. Although it is not unanimous, consensus has emerged about four broad principles: (1) all clinicians should treat all their patients with the best available resources of modern medicine unless there are powerful reasons to do otherwise; (2) in the United States today, any mentally competent and informed adult can voluntarily refuse to accept any medical intervention even if that refusal results in his or her death; (3) parents have neither a moral right nor a legal right to refuse modern medicine as such or blood transfusions for their children; (4) subtle clinical discretion is permissible in a very few cases when a child or minor is almost an adult who understandingly refuses an intervention as his or her own decision.

In a different way, though, the four movements represent the common nineteenth-century American openness to bold experimentation with new interpretations of scripture and new ways of being Christian – a tradition that has continued in manifold ways throughout the twentieth century and into the twenty-first.

Conclusion

Over the last 2,000 years, Christianity has made many twists and turns while never entirely losing its own identity. At this time in the United States, Christianity is a conglomerate of diverse theologies and historical expressions with Roman Catholics, Orthodox Christians, Evangelical Protestants, and Mainline Protestants aligning themselves in different ways from one issue to another. For the most part, although there are important exceptions, Catholics, Evangelical Protestants, and the Orthodox tend to represent the "conservative" wing of Christianity, while Mainline Protestants tend to occupy the "liberal" wing. This pattern is evident and persistent in the relationships between these Christian groups and health and healing. Despite stark differences on a number of theological and bioethical issues, however, Christians are still able to find connectedness with each other through their common commitment to understanding and applying the Bible, common faith in Jesus, and mutual engagement in the world for positive transformation.

Table 13.1 Dos and don'ts: Latter-day Saints

Dos	Don'ts
1. Be respectful of the patient's dietary specifications (no caffeine).	1. Do not speak condescendingly of the patient's or Latter-day Saints' view on diet.
2. Involve the family in decision making.	2. The preferred name of the group is "Latter-day Saint," rather than Mormon, though the latter is not an offensive term.
3. Ask if the patient wishes to see a Latter-day Saint leader.	

Table 13.2 Dos and don'ts: Seventh-day Adventists

Dos	Don'ts
1. Be respectful of the patient's dietary specifications (often no meat or fish). 2. Be respectful of Sabbath considerations. 3. Facilitate the patient's wish to use a more natural means to the degree that it is possible. 4. Facilitate the patient's desire for prayer and anointing by an Adventist pastor or elder.	1. Do not speak condescendingly of the patient's or Adventists' view on diet and Sabbath-keeping.

Table 13.3 Dos and don'ts: Christian Scientists

Dos	Don'ts
1. Explain fully and clearly the physiological effects and implications of each procedure. 2. Ask to what degree the patient wishes to receive medical care and drugs and respect his/her right of refusal. 3. Find out what arrangements the patient and his/her family has made for the dying. 4. Help locate a Christian Science practitioner for prayers of healing. 5. Allow time for personal prayer.	1. Do not speak condescendingly of the patient's or Christian Scientists' suspicion toward medical care. 2. Do not insist on specific care that the patient is uncomfortable with. 3. Do not make any medical decisions, even simple ones, without explaining everything fully.

Table 13.4 Dos and don'ts: Jehovah's Witnesses

Dos	Don'ts
1. Respect the patient's desire to avoid blood transfusion and storage. 2. Explain fully and clearly how the blood will be used and disposed of when it is drawn. 3. Work with the Hospital Information Services of Jehovah's Witnesses' Watch Tower Society if bloodless surgery is an option. 4. Be sensitive to the fact that Jehovah's Witnesses do not involve themselves in politics or celebrate holidays, including birthdays.	1. Do not speak condescendingly of the patient's or Jehovah's Witnesses' view on blood. 2. Do not make any medical decisions, even simple ones, without explaining everything fully.

Case study #1

Sirya is a 17½-year-old girl in need of oral surgery to remove all four of her wisdom teeth. She and her parents both want to have it done under general anesthesia in the surgical suite at their local 400-bed hospital. Sirya is anxious about the procedure and wants to be "out of it" with the use of general anesthesia.

When the anesthesiologist met with Sirya and her parents they were surprised at facing the question of consent for reception of blood products if the need arose during the procedure. Sirya and her parents are members of the Jehovah's Witness faith and do not accept blood products.

The anesthesiologist was very understanding and professional in his response, in part, because he has family who are members of the Jehovah's Witness faith. Nonetheless, he was firm in his position that he would not do the anesthesia work for the procedure without their consent to receive blood. He even surveyed his colleagues to see if any of them would do the procedure, but a full week later none of them had agreed to do it.

At this point, Sirya was ready to consent to the blood products but her parents continued to refuse. Instead, the parents insisted upon a care conference with the hospital's administration, Risk Management representative, ethics consultant, and compliance officer to see if there was something they could do to bypass the anesthesiologist's hesitancy. Unfortunately, there was not. Frustrated, Sirya and her parents left the hospital.

Questions for reflection

1. Is it professionally appropriate for an anesthesiologist to refuse involvement in this case?
2. Is there some sort of special exception that can be made for Jehovah's Witnesses to receive blood in emergency situations?
3. Was it right that the parents insisted that Sirya refuse blood products, or should she have been given the option to choose for herself?
4. Why couldn't the hospital and those involved in the care conference override the anesthesiologist's decision?

Submitted by Mark F. Carr

Case study #2

At a 450-bed hospital in a large city, several nurses on the medical rehab unit complained to their manager about a co-worker who had every Saturday off for religious purposes. The staff members felt that the distribution of staffing was unfair as it required that the remainder of the staff take on proportionally more Saturday shifts. Further, they did not understand why their colleague would require Saturday for religious observance since he made it obvious to everyone that he was Christian.

The nurse manager discussed the concerns with the Adventist staff member and asked for clarification regarding his request for religious accommodations. The nurse manager echoed the staff's concerns that this was an inequitable arrangement. The nurse explained that he was a Seventh-day Adventist, and his faith required that he observe the Sabbath on Saturday.

Questions for reflection

1. What religious beliefs underlie this Seventh-day Adventist nurse's request? Are there any official Church statements about healthcare personnel working on Sabbath?

2. Do you believe the situation is equitable? Why or why not?
3. Given that Seventh-day Adventist operate hundreds of hospitals with plenty of Church members working at them on Saturdays, how ought the manager respond to the Adventist nurse's request?
4. What are the nurse's rights in this scenario?

Submitted by Joset Brown

Glossary

Latter-day Saints

Book of Mormon A book believed to be a revelation of Jesus Christ that contains stories of God's people in North America throughout the centuries.
Endowment Ritual consisting of symbolic acts and covenants that is performed in a Latter-day Saint temple.
Joseph Smith (1805–1844) The founder and first prophet of the Church of Jesus Christ of Latter-day Saints.
Temple Recommend A certificate given to Latter-day Saints by church leadership for entrance to the temple. It is given only after the member is able to show worthiness by answering a series of questions.

Seventh-day Adventists

Ellen White (1827–1915) One of the co-founders of the Seventh-day Adventist Church.
Great Disappointment A term used to describe what took place on October 22, 1844, among those who awaited the return of Jesus Christ that day.
Health message Adventist teaching about the connection between the body, mind, and spirit and the importance of complete wholeness as part of one's preparation for the second coming of Christ.
Vegetarianism Adventists recommend vegetarianism as the ideal dietary choice. It stems from their emphasis on health as part of the call to a life of wholeness.

Christian Scientists

Divine Mind Another name for God. Used very often due to Christian Scientists' emphasis on the mental and the spiritual as the only reality.
Mary Baker Eddy (1821–1910) The founder of Christian Science.
Practitioners Individuals who practice healing through prayer according to the principles of Christian Science. Qualified practitioners are typically listed in the *Christian Science Journal* and www.spirituality.com.
Science and Health A book written by Maker Baker Eddy and published originally in 1875 and expanded in 1883 with "Key to the Scriptures." Considered an inspired book that stands on equal footing with the Bible, it provides a description of the principles of Christian Science.

Jehovah's Witnesses

Bloodless surgery A method of surgery without the use of another person's blood; some may choose to use their own blood in a bloodless surgery.

Charles Taze Russell (1852–1916) Founder of the Jehovah's Witnesses movement.

Kingdom Hall Meeting place of the Jehovah's Witnesses, the external appearance of which is similar to a modest Christian church yet without any of the typical external symbols.

Watch Tower Society The central administrative organization of Jehovah's Witnesses.

Note

All quotations from the Hebrew scriptures, Torah and Ketuvim, are translations of the author.

1 Julius J. Nam, the original author of this chapter, was unable to be involved in the update for this third edition. We appreciate David R. Larson for his help updating it.

Bibliography

Church of Jesus Christ of Latter-day Saints (2022). *Worldwide statistics*. Churchofjesuschrist.org. https://newsroom.churchofjesuschrist.org/facts-and-statistics

Eddy, Mary Baker (1907) *Science and Health with Key to the Scriptures*. Available online: www.marybakereddylibrary.org/research/the-development-of-the-scientific-statement-of-being

Jehovah's Witnesses (2014) *Jehovah's Witnesses Reach Membership Milestones*. Watch Tower Bible and Tract Society of Pennsylvania. www.jw.org/en/jehovahs-witnesses/activities/ministry/how-many-jehovahs-witnesses-2014/

Jehovah's Witnesses (2022) How Many of Jehovah's Witnesses Are There Worldwide? Watch Tower Bible and Tract Society of Pennsylvania. www.jw.org/en/jehovahs-witnesses/faq/how-many-jw-members/#?insight[search_id]=95febd96-8c84-4035-9fe6-a5c057ceaf0a

New Revised Standard Version Bible (Anglicized) With Apocrypha (1995) New York: Oxford University Press.

Russell, Charles Taze (1886) *Millenial Dawn*, vol. 1, The Plan of the Ages. Alleghany, PA: Tower Publishing Co. pp. 267–268. Available online: https://books.google.com/books?id=ADUQA AAAYAAJ&pg=PA267&dq#v=onepage&q&f=false

Seventh-day Adventist Church (2015) *2015 Annual Statistical Report: 151st Report of the General Conference Seventh-day Adventists for 2013 and 2014*. http://documents.adventistarchives.org/Statistics/ASR/ASR2015.pdf

Seventh-day Adventist Church (2021) *Seventh-day Adventist World Church Statistics 2021*. www.adventist.org/statistics/

Smith, Joseph Jr. (n.d.) *The Church of Jesus Christ of Latter-day Saints*. Doctrines and Covenants, Section 137:7-9. www.churchofjesuschrist.org/study/scriptures/dc-testament/dc/137?lang=eng

The Christian Science Journal (2022) *The Christian Science Journal Directory of Professional Services and Church Information*. https://journal.christianscience.com/

White, Ellen G. (1914) *The Advent Review and Sabbath Herald*, vol. 91, no. 18, p. 4. https://documents.adventistarchives.org/Periodicals/RH/RH19140430-V91-18.pdf

14 Conclusion

Mark F. Carr

The prevailing posture in Western medicine is to search for physical explanations of illness and diseases – to identify the virus, to locate the tumor, to search for the specific neuronal connection. Ever a quest to find and destroy that which ails us, always seeking the cure. These chapters exploring health and disease from the perspectives of world religions remind us that illness is a universal human experience. Illness affects the physical, mental, emotional, and spiritual realities of all human persons. Conversely, we learn from the wisdom of these religions that the way we see reality, the way we interpret events, and the way we connect with each other and with divinity can positively influence the way we experience illness and health. If we are unable to overcome the illness or find the cure, how might religion and spirituality help us cope?

Healthcare providers have come to the important realization that the way one lives out religious beliefs profoundly influences the experience of illness and the process of healing. We better understand variations in the way people interpret cancer, kidney disease, heart failure, and many other diseases, and the way belief systems affect health and the treatment process. Understanding the believer's interpretation of illness and health necessitates careful consideration in treating patients from various faith traditions because it is ultimately the patients' religious understanding of the meaning in life that defines health and wellness for them. Lack of understanding patient belief systems can lead to deterioration of their health because it may create internal conflicts that generate negative thoughts, emotions, and spiritual experiences, ultimately impeding the healing process.

Understanding the role religion plays in healthcare may generate different questions for healthcare professionals to ponder – questions regarding the validity of various faith traditions and the different approaches they can (and ought to) take toward other religions. Initially, there are two options for us as caregivers: open and closed. One may either be open to the possibility that true and genuine religious beliefs and experiences are possible in more than one religion or one may be closed to that possibility. For those who belong to the latter group, there is only one valid religion – their own.

On the other hand, those who are open to seeing other religions as valid have further questions to consider. Are all religions equally valid? Are there degrees of validity? Are there any objective criteria with which to evaluate religions? If so, what are they and who sets these criteria? If not, are all evaluations of religion ultimately subjective? For some, while they recognize that other religions can offer valid pathways to the Divine, they view their own as the definitive religion. Judging the validity of religions often revolves around

DOI: 10.4324/9781003288862-14

certain general criteria, such as recognition of the Divine, practice of distinct rituals, ethical behaviors, the history of its founders, their stories, and those who followed.

Perhaps the most prevalent stance toward the other is to simply engage *without judgment*. Humans are simply religious beings. This approach stresses dialogue among religions and mutual learning among the followers of the world's religions – including those who do not identify with a specific religion: the "nones," agnostics, and atheists.

Regardless of the approach you may take – personally or corporately within one's own faith tradition – the posture motivating the editors and authors of this book is one of openness, understanding, and respect. In an increasingly shrinking world where religions, denominations, sects, and groups interface with one another daily, it is important – regardless of how one views other religions – to understand and respect others. Understanding and respect do not equal agreement or even appreciation. But they lead to more informed interactions that make for friendlier neighborhoods, healthier societies, and a more peaceful world – and in your professional sphere, more compassionate patient care.

In addition to how we interact with those of other religious traditions, we trust that in your work as a healthcare practitioner your education about the religions in this book will enhance your professionalism and compassion. As noted in the preface, when individual practitioners and entire facilities pay attention to the religious practices and needs of patients, everyone is benefited. The individual patient's healing encounter is enhanced, the practitioner experiences a more fulfilling encounter with the patient, and the facility itself incurs greater respect and credibility in the local community it serves.

As Western medical science evolves along its technological path, it has and will likely continue to learn to be more open and appreciative of other perspectives on what it means to be healthy. Rather than simply being purveyors of medical technology, healthcare professionals of all sorts may learn to be healers. Some less technical, more traditional, and religious methods of addressing human health and illness may enhance Western medicine rather than clash with it. We hope that clashes can be avoided as we learn more about the traditional and religious methods of handling illness. Yet we also want to urge practitioners not to simply accept each and every religious or traditional method. Some methods may in fact harm patients rather than help them. But it is only a discerning practitioner, one who has taken the effort to learn of the other, who will be able to address the healing encounter with balance and equanimity.

Like the healing enterprise, religion is not staid. Religion and its traditions are ever evolving, always adjusting to the cultures they encounter and help to shape. Some of the issues addressed in this text are relatively new and troublesome for religion to deal with. The advance of medical technology brings difficult questions of life-sustaining healthcare, reproductive assistance, abortion, and even diet. This list can be lengthened, but the point is that religion and culture (and thus medical science) are inextricably connected with each other. They continually modify each other and so it should be no surprise that medicine and religion will do the same thing. While existential questions of life and death remain the domain of faith and religion, medical technologies and cultural acceptance of these technologies change the way we discuss life and death, even in religious circles. Take, for instance, the notion that life begins at the moment of conception. For millennia, prior to microscopic means of watching the blending of DNA, religion recognized the profundity and sacredness of human reproduction with no specific, scientific knowledge of conception. Today, medical science can detail for us every second of the process. As it turns out, there is no "moment" of conception that delineates between life and no life. When a religious leader stands and speaks of the moment of conception and a medical researcher stands and uses the same phrase, we see that the two may be speaking of the same event with quite different emphases.

The same can be said of the matter of death. Prior to the technical capability to measure activity in the brain, a person was considered dead when the heart stopped pumping and the person stopped breathing. Religion has always had something to say about death and yet, in this day when machines and drugs can keep these functions active, we wrestle with what it means to be "brain dead." Religion continues to be relevant even in the face of appropriate, changing scientific definitions of life and death. Science and religion interact and influence each other.

Finally, our introductory chapter author, Ernest J. Bursey, suggested that the readers of this text would benefit from the purposeful encounter with someone of a different religion. Have you done the same over the course of reading this text? In full agreement, the authors and editors want to end our text with a reminder that, by engaging the Other in meaningful conversation, you and your healthcare practice will be enhanced and enriched.

Index

Note: Page numbers in *italic* refers to Tables.

Printed in the United States
by Baker & Taylor Publisher Services